O P L

OXFORD PSYCHIATRY LIBRARY

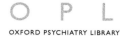

Managing Negative Symptoms of Schizophrenia

T0177595

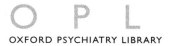

OXFORD PSYCHIATRY LIBRARY

Managing Negative Symptoms of Schizophrenia

Edited by

István Bitter

Professor of Psychiatry, Department of Psychiatry and
Psychotherapy, Semmelweis University, Budapest, Hungary

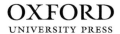

OXFORD
UNIVERSITY PRESS

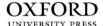

UNIVERSITY PRESS

Great Clarendon Street, Oxford, OX2 6DP,
United Kingdom

Oxford University Press is a department of the University of Oxford.
It furthers the University's objective of excellence in research, scholarship,
and education by publishing worldwide. Oxford is a registered trade mark of
Oxford University Press in the UK and in certain other countries

First Edition published in 2020

Impression: 2

Published in the United States of America by Oxford University Press
198 Madison Avenue, New York, NY 10016, United States of America

British Library Cataloguing in Publication Data

Data available

Library of Congress Control Number: 2019957196

ISBN 978–0–19–884012–1

Printed and bound by
CPI Group (UK) Ltd, Croydon, CR0 4YY

Foreword

Schizophrenia has a worldwide prevalence of between 0.4 per cent and 1.4 per cent. Out of this group of patients up to 90 per cent experience negative symptoms. Negative symptoms have been recognized as key components of schizophrenia since the first descriptions of this mental disorder by Emil Kraepelin and later on by Eugen Bleuler. About 20–30 per cent of these patients show several domains of negative symptoms characteristic for this group, having an increased risk for enduring symptomatology and unfavourable outcome. However, the progress in the development of innovative treatments has so far been slow and negative symptoms represent an unmet need in the care of subjects with schizophrenia.

This has triggered a growing interest in this sub-syndrome of schizophrenia, undermined by the evidence of the strong relationship of negative symptoms with low remission rates, poor real-life functioning, and quality of life. In the light of the strong impact on functional outcome and the burden on patients, relatives, and healthcare systems, negative symptoms have become a key target in the search for new therapeutic tools. It is therefore imperative to focus on the conceptualization, descriptions, and treatment of negative symptoms. *Managing Negative Symptoms in Schizophrenia* does exactly that: the authors of this book pay particular attention to the contemporary research into negative symptoms, which has produced many interesting new findings. However, the interpretation of these new findings has been controversial, and this book devotes particular attention to the inclusion of the varied views of different research groups on current issues about negative symptoms in schizophrenia, with opinions partly corresponding to but also showing a rich diversity in their views. István Bitter's primary ambition during the writing and editing of this book was to focus on 'real-world' patients and to present material which can help improve the care for patients with negative symptoms of schizophrenia. The authors of this book have accomplished this task in an exceptional way.

Peter Falkai
Munich, December 2019

Preface

Recent years have witnessed an increased interest in negative symptoms, which have been considered to be the fundamental or core symptoms of schizophrenia. Contemporary research into negative symptoms has produced new findings; however, their interpretation has been controversial. This book devotes particular attention to the inclusion of the views of different research groups on current issues in this field.

The chapter contributors to this book present a variety of opinions about negative symptoms in schizophrenia. Whilst these opinions are partly corresponding, we can find a rich diversity in their views, including, but not limited to, answers to the following questions: which signs and symptoms belong to the negative symptom domain in schizophrenia? How can we differentiate primary negative symptoms of schizophrenia from the clinically identical secondary negative symptoms which are associated, for example, with other mental disorders (e.g. substance use), with other symptoms of schizophrenia (e.g. depression), with social isolation, and with poverty (e.g. lack of opportunities)?

Current research is focusing on primary persistent negative symptoms, even though negative symptoms are very rarely present in schizophrenia without other symptoms (e.g. positive symptoms, anxiety, depression, extrapyramidal symptoms). Despite the frequent coexistence of these symptoms, their relationship, and especially their long-term association, has rarely been the subject of research. Most of the scales on negative symptoms are based on observer rating. The patient's self-assessments and self-experiences (including the so-called basic symptoms) have been vastly overlooked both in research and clinical work. The individual signs and symptoms are of utmost importance in the search for biological markers. Total scores of negative symptom scales are useful in clinical studies measuring changes of the severity of symptoms from baseline to endpoint. However, reducing multiple items/symptoms to a single score is associated with loss of valuable information, which may be essential for research into the pathophysiology and aetiology of schizophrenia.

The above mentioned topics and questions have been addressed in this book along with the current consensus on the five domains of negative symptoms. The different viewpoints and constructs described by the chapter contributors are complementary rather than exclusive. Their knowledge helps to improve the diagnosis and treatment of negative symptoms and contribute to the progress of research in this field.

The two chapters in this book that focus on the treatment of negative symptoms in schizophrenia support clinical practice with evidence-based recommendations both for pharmacological and psychosocial treatments. We have been stricter with recommending pharmacological treatments than psychosocial therapies, as the benefit–risk ratio is questionable or even unfavourable for some off-label pharmacological treatment attempts reported in the literature. Whilst some of them merit further research, we definitively would not like to encourage treatment practices without sufficient evidence for a favourable benefit–risk ratio.

My primary consideration during editing this book was to focus on 'real world' patients, and to present material in this small book, which can help improve the care for patients with negative symptoms of schizophrenia.

István Bitter
Budapest, September 2019

Contents

Abbreviations

ACIPS	Anticipatory and Consummatory Interpersonnal Pleasure Scale
AD	antidepressants
ADHD	attention deficit hyperactivity disorder
AES-S	Self-reported Apathy Evaluation Scale
AMPA	α-amino-3-hydroxy-5-methyl-4-isoxazolepropionic acid
ASA	acetylsalicylic acid
BNSS	Brief Negative Symptom Scale
BPRS	Brief Psychiatric Rating Scale
BS	basic symptoms
BSA	broad-spectrum agent
BSABS	Bonn Scale for the Assessment of Basic Symptoms
CAINS	Clinical Assessment Interview for Negative Symptoms
CANSAS	Collaboration to Advance Negative Symptom Assessment in Schizophrenia
CAPE	Community Assessment of Psychic Experiences
CBTp	Cognitive Behavioural Therapy for Psychosis
CDRS	Calgary Depression Rating Scale
CDSS	Calgary Depression Scale for Schizophrenia
CHMP	Committee for Medicinal Products for Human Use
COGDIS	Cognitive Disturbances
COPER	Cognitive-Perceptive Basic Symptoms
COX-2	cyclo-oxygenase-2
DA	dopamine
DHEA	dehydroepiandrosterone
DLPFC	dorsolateral prefrontal cortex
EMA	European Medicines Agency
EPS	extrapyramidal symptoms
FCQ	Frankfurt Complaint Questionnaire
FDA	Food and Drug Administration
FGA	first-generation antipsychotics
GABAA	γ-aminobutyric acid A
GLU	glutamatergic medications
ICD-10	International Statistical Classification of Diseases and Health Problems, 10th revision
IS	Insight scale

MAP–SR	Motivation and Pleasure Scale–Self-Report
MATRICS	Measurement and Treatment Research to Improve Cognition in Schizophrenia
NAC	N-acetyl-cysteine
NIMH	National Institute of Mental Health
NMDA	N-Methyl-D-Aspartate Acid
NSA	Negative Symptom Assessment
NSAID	nonsteroidal anti-inflammatory drug
PANSS	Positive and Negative Syndrome Scale
PAS	Physical Anhedonia Scale
PCA	principal component analysis
PNS	persistent negative symptoms
RCTs	randomized controlled trials
ROC	receiver operating characteristic
R-SAS	Revised Social Anhedonia Scale
rTMS	repetitive transcranial magnetic stimulation
SA	standard antipsychotic agent
SAAS	Self-Assessment Anhedonia Scale
SANS	Scale for the Assessment of Negative Symptoms
SAS	Social Anhedonia Scale
SD	standard deviation
SEDS	Subjective Experience of Deficits in Schizophrenia
SENS	Subjective Experience of Negative Symptoms
SGA	second-generation antipsychotics
SDSS	Subjective Deficit Syndrome Scale
SIPS	Structured Interview for Psychosis-Risk Syndromes
SMD	standardized mean difference
SNS	Self-evaluation of Negative Symptoms
SPI-A	Schizophrenia Proneness Instruments-Adult version
SPI-CY	Schizophrenia Proneness Instruments-Child and Youth version
SSRI	selective serotonin reuptake inhibitor
TAU	treatment as usual
tDCS	transcranial direct current stimulation
TEPS	Temporal Experience of Pleasure Scale
UHR	ultra-high risk
WHO	World Health Organization

Contributors

István Bitter, Professor of Psychiatry, Department of Psychiatry and Psychotherapy, Semmelweis University, Budapest, Hungary

Pál Czobor, Associate Professor, Department of Psychiatry and Psychotherapy, Semmelweis University, Budapest, Hungary

Sonia Dollfus, Professor of Psychiatry, Head of Department of Mental Health at the CHU, Psychiatry Department of the University Hospital of Caen Normandy, Caen, France

Dmitry Romanov, Professor of Department, Department of Psychiatry and Psychosomatics, Sechenov First Moscow State Medical University (Sechenov University) and Department of Boundary Conditions and Psychosomatic Disorders Mental Health Research Center, Moscow, Russia

Mark Savill, Researcher, Department of Psychiatry, UCSF, San Francisco, California, USA

Frauke Schultze-Lutter, Assistant Professor, Senior Researcher, Head of the "Early detection" Unit and the FEZ, Department of Psychiatry and Psychotherapy, Medical Faculty of the Heinrich-Heine University Düsseldorf, Düsseldorf, Germany

Anatoly Smulevich, Professor, Academic of of the Russian Academy of Sciences, Head of Department, Department of Psychiatry and Psychosomatics, Sechenov First Moscow State Medical University (Sechenov University) and Department of Boundary Conditions and Psychosomatic Disorders, Mental Health Research Center, Moscow, Russia

Anais Vandevelde, Psychiatrist, Health Mental Department at the CHU, University of Caen Normandie, Caen, France

CHAPTER 1

Definitions and measurement of negative symptoms in schizophrenia

István Bitter

KEY POINTS

- Negative symptoms are present in the broadly defined behaviour and also in the subjective experiences of the patients with schizophrenia.
- Persistent primary negative symptoms are considered to be part of the schizophrenia disease process and represent an unmet need for treatment.
- Secondary negative symptoms associated with positive symptoms of schizophrenia, other mental disorders (e.g. depression, substance abuse), extrapyramidal symptoms, social deprivation, etc., should be evaluated and treated.
- Negative symptoms can be reliable evaluated and measured.
- Validated rating scales help in the clinical evaluation and research of negative symptoms.

1.1 Introduction

Schizophrenia is a mental disorder that typically first presents in patients during their late teens to early thirties and is often associated with poor social and occupational functioning, and high disability and mortality rates. It is characterized by symptoms that can be broadly described as negative and positive.

Positive symptoms of schizophrenia are, for example, hallucinations, disorganized thinking, and delusions. Positive symptoms are usually well recognized by healthcare professionals as well as lay persons. Current treatment methods are generally effective in the management of positive symptoms.

Negative symptoms of schizophrenia represent deficits in different domains, such as loss or diminution in emotions, thinking, and movement. Examples of negative symptoms are anhedonia, avolition (lack of motivation/will to accomplish tasks or even to initiate them), blunted affect, and poverty of speech. The concepts, definitions, and measurement methods of negative symptoms have large heterogeneity as compared to positive symptoms. Primary negative symptoms have been considered to be part of the disease process in schizophrenia, while secondary negative symptoms are associated with well-defined aetiologies, for example positive symptoms, comorbid psychiatric or neurological diseases (e.g. depression or extrapyramidal diseases, respectively), side effects of medications, or social deprivation. If we do not consider cognitive symptoms as part of the negative symptom domain then patients with negative symptoms have more cognitive symptoms than patients without them. Negative symptoms are often not well recognized and primary negative symptoms do not respond at all or respond poorly to most available treatments. One out of four or five patients with schizophrenia has primary persisting negative symptoms, which would 'merit therapeutic intervention' (Kirkpatrick, Fenton, Carpenter, et al. 2006). Seven per cent of first-episode patients had persistent negative symptoms, which were associated with poorer psychopathological and functional outcomes after one year (Galderisi, Mucci, Bitter, et al. 2013).

Negative symptoms have been considered as the core of the psychopathology or fundamental symptoms in schizophrenia. Since negative symptoms are associated with poor functioning and outcome in schizophrenia, their recognition, proper evaluation, and treatment are of great importance.

The descriptions of the signs and symptoms of schizophrenia have always included negative symptoms, however the definition of negative symptoms has been changing over time. Kraepelin described—partly based on earlier works—both cognitive (progressive dementia) and negative symptoms (e.g. patients became indifferent, apathetic, mute, or gave sparse answers, have lost their 'own will') as characteristic for dementia praecox (Kraepelin, 1904). Bleuler described negative symptoms, the famous 'four As' as fundamental symptoms of schizophrenia: associative loosening, affective blunting, autism, and ambivalence. He considered hallucinations and delusions (the positive symptoms) as accessory symptoms of schizophrenia (Bleuler, 1983). Jackson has been credited with the conceptualization of negative symptoms of neurological and psychiatric diseases. He considered 'evolution' (brain activity) to be the source of positive symptoms (e.g. motor symptoms of an epileptic 'fit' or disturbances of perception in a mental illness) and negative symptoms to be the consequences of 'dissolution' (decrease of functions) of the brain. He wrote: 'Negative and positive mental symptoms are for us only signs of what is not going on, or of what is going on wrong in the highest sensori-motor centres.' (Jackson, 1887). Jackson also gave examples of the coexistence of positive and negative symptoms (e.g. 'dissolution' of prefrontal lobe activity reflected by motor paresis and 'evolution' of temporal lobe activity reflected by illusions after an epileptic seizure). The analysis of the chronological pattern of the coexistence and the relationship of positive and negative symptoms is very important for the evaluation and understanding of negative symptoms in schizophrenia. Chapter 3 of this book by Smulevich and Romanov gives an overview of the complexity of the long-term course of various negative syndrome phenotypes. Primary negative symptoms may be present with positive symptoms, cognitive symptoms, secondary negative symptoms, and other symptoms that are classified as 'general psychopathology' symptoms in schizophrenia (e.g. depression).

The work of Schneider in the middle of the twentieth century changed the focus from negative to positive symptoms in the diagnostic criteria for schizophrenia (Schneider, 1980). He considered the group of 'first-rank symptoms' typical for schizophrenia, while the 'second-rank symptoms' were less important for its diagnosis. Both the first- and second-rank symptoms are positive symptoms. First-rank symptoms include: voices making comments, voices heard inside the head, voices talking to each other, thoughts becoming audible, the belief that thoughts are being inserted into or removed from the head, thoughts are being broadcast, real/true hallucinations (hallucinations having an 'objective reality' with delusional interpretation), and the belief that thoughts, feelings, and actions will be controlled from outside the individual. Examples of second-rank symptoms are: non-auditory hallucinations and paranoid delusions. Both currently widely used diagnostic systems in psychiatry, the International Classification of Diseases 10th revision (and the upcoming 11th revision) by the World Health Organization and the Diagnostic and Statistical Manual, 5th edition by the American Psychiatric Association, rely heavily on the presence of positive symptoms for the diagnosis of schizophrenia.

In the 1980s a revival of interest in negative symptoms led to new research, which resulted in new definitions (e.g. deficit schizophrenia) and in more specific rating scales for the evaluation of negative symptoms (e.g. the Scale for the Assessment of Negative Symptoms (SANS) and the Positive and Negative Syndrome Scale (PANSS)), which will be discussed later in this chapter; SANS is included in the Appendix of this book.

A project called 'Measurement and Treatment Research to Improve Cognition in Schizophrenia' (MATRICS) initiated by the US National Institute of Mental Health (NIMH) led to a consensus conference on negative symptoms in schizophrenia in 2005. As a result of this meeting the 'NIMH-MATRICS consensus statement on negative symptoms' was published (Kirkpatrick, et al. 2006). The participants of the conference achieved consensus on eleven points which have served as guidance for further research. One of the points included the five domains of negative symptoms as they have been currently understood: blunted affect, alogia, asociality, anhedonia, and avolition (the five 'As'). The participants also agreed that 'Negative symptoms and cognitive impairments represent separate domains', and 'Negative symptoms constitute a distinct therapeutic indication area'. It was also noted that the interaction and potential overlap of negative and cognitive symptoms warrants further research.

Both the European (European Medicines Agency, EMA) and the US (Food and Drug Administration, FDA) regulatory agencies contributed to the definition of negative symptoms and to the development of clinical trial methodology for negative symptoms in schizophrenia. The viewpoint of the FDA (Laughren and Levin, 2006) will be addressed in Chapter 5, written by Czobor and Bitter; some specifics of the EMA viewpoint (EMA, 2013) will be discussed in this chapter.

1.2 Evaluation of the negative symptoms in schizophrenia

Negative symptoms can be evaluated by an observer (e.g. psychiatrist, psychologist, other healthcare professional, relative, friend, teacher) or by the patients themselves. Some subjective experiences of patients with schizophrenia may be part of the negative syndrome and the subjective experiences can be reliable measured (Bitter, Jaeger, Agdeppa, et al. 1989). Self-evaluation of negative symptoms and basic disturbances and self-evaluation instruments are discussed in Chapter 2 and Chapter 4 of this book, written by Schultze-Lutter and Dollfus and Vandevelde, respectively. The importance of separating the expressive and experiential domains of negative symptoms has also been reflected in the design of the Clinical Assessment Interview for Negative Symptoms (CAINS) (Horan, Kring, Gur, et al. 2011).

The evaluation of each negative symptom is based on a definition of what the clinician (or researcher in case of a clinical study) is looking for and different definitions and names may exist for the same symptom. Different authors and schools of thought, as well as diagnostic scales, do not always agree on symptom definition. In this chapter we try to include and define a broad range of negative symptoms and provide the different names for the same (or similar) symptoms. However, it is also important to emphasize that current evidence supports the five factor/symptom construct of negative symptoms.

Information for the evaluation of negative symptoms can be gathered from all available sources, however some symptoms can only be observed during the interview (e.g. lack of spontaneity and flow of conversation). The evaluation of other symptoms (e.g. social withdrawal) should include or even should be exclusively based on information from other observers, such as family members and other healthcare professionals.

The usual *time frame* for the cross-sectional evaluation of negative symptoms in clinical practice and in most clinical trials is one week (i.e. the week before the clinical interview). Persistent or enduring negative symptoms are defined as negative symptoms lasting at least 6 months (based on the cited EMA guidelines) or 12 months (based on the definition of *deficit schizophrenia*). Negative symptoms frequently precede the onset of the first episode with positive symptoms in schizophrenia. Research into subjective experiences contributed to the improvement of early intervention programmes for patients at high risk for psychosis/schizophrenia and to a better understanding of primary versus secondary negative symptoms.

1.2.1 Negative symptoms of schizophrenia: list of symptoms and symptom definitions

Affective flattening or blunting—paucity or lack of gestures including hypomimia (decreased, or even lack of, facial expression); monotony (lack of modulation) in speech; lack of affective response (e.g. no smiling in response to another person);

poor eye contact. The lack of experience of any negative emotion (lack of distress) even in unpleasant situations may be part of affective flattening or blunting.

Motor retardation and hypomimia are also observed—as secondary negative symptoms—in depression during schizophrenia and Parkinson syndrome caused by various antipsychotics used for the treatment of schizophrenia.

Alogia—poverty of the amount and/or the content of the speech; short answers to questions, flow of discussion interrupted with pauses, the interviewer has to ask many questions to keep the conversation going. It is important that some languages/psychiatrists use the term alogia as a synonym for 'illogical', not as a change (decrease) in quantity of speech and its content, but as a qualitative change; the lack of logical thinking, which is a positive symptom, also called illogicality (e.g. in SANS) or illogical thinking/speech. Slow speech is also a symptom of other conditions (e.g. depression, Parkinson syndrome, sedation).

Asociality—being isolated, having little or no interest in having friends, not going out, not being involved in 'social life'. This term is used today instead of 'autism' which was introduced as one of the fundamental symptoms of schizophrenia by Bleuler. Bleuler considered autism in schizophrenia as withdrawal from real life into the 'internal life' of the patients. It is important to differentiate this term from 'antisocial' or 'anti-sociality'. The term 'emotional withdrawal' combines asociality and affective flattening/blunting as causes of detachment from persons and events in the real world. Asociality is present both in the behaviour and subjective experiences of the patients (feels fine alone, no desire to have more contacts or to get closer to people).

Anhedonia—Gard and colleagues (2007) found anticipatory but not a consummatory pleasure deficit in schizophrenia. Consummatory anhedonia describes the lack of enjoyment from current activities, while anticipatory anhedonia describes the lack of anticipation of pleasure from future activities. This subdivision contributed to the understanding of earlier controversial findings about anhedonia in schizophrenia: patients reported more anhedonia than healthy controls during interviews, however they reported similar to healthy control levels of pleasure to stimuli in experimental settings. Based on this subdivision of anhedonia in addition to exploring the frequency and the intensity of pleasurable activities during the last week, *anticipation of intensity of future expected pleasure* should also be explored in different areas, for example work and school (if applicable), social contacts, positive physical feelings.

Anhedonia can also be caused by antipsychotics—especially by some first-generation antipsychotics—which are dopamine receptor antagonists inhibiting the reward system.

Avolition—earlier descriptions also used the words abulia/hypobulia referring to the lack/decrease of wilful initiation of activities, such as any movement or talking with others. This symptom may lead to neglecting personal care, hygiene, and grooming. The term asthenia was used to describe lack/loss of energy (anergia), mental and physical fatigue. Avolition includes both the behavioural manifestations (performed activities) and the experiences of the patients (thinking/motivation about activities;

missing activities). In German the term 'disorders of drive' ('Antriebstörungen') also describes the lack of or diminished drive.

Avolition, emotional detachment, apathy, and lack of drive all contribute to *passive/apathetic social withdrawal*, which is one of the negative items in PANSS. Avolition is also a frequent symptom of depression.

A number of negative symptoms, which are part of various rating scales are currently considered as *cognitive symptoms*, for example *stereotyped thinking, impairment in abstract thinking*, and *disturbances of attention*.

Disturbances of attention in schizophrenia have been associated with both negative and positive symptoms. *Disturbances of social attention or social inattentiveness*, a symptom which has been classified as a negative item in SANS, is an item which is difficult to interpret. A patient with schizophrenia may have well-documented impairment of emotion perception—including increased responsivity to fearful faces (Komlósi, Csukly, Stefanics, et al. 2013)—which has been linked to temporal lobe ('social brain') dysfunctions and to antipsychotics to some degree as well. Social inattentiveness may be linked to the impairment of emotion perception and may contribute to a number of negative symptoms such as affective flattening or blunting, asociality, and emotional withdrawal. However, the MATRIX-NIMH consensus concluded that social cognition, as usually defined, is not part of the negative symptom construct.

1.3 Classification of negative symptoms

1.3.1 Primary and secondary negative symptoms

Primary negative symptoms are considered to be part of the disease process in schizophrenia. As mentioned earlier, secondary negative symptoms are causally associated with well-defined aetiologies, for example positive symptoms or comorbid psychiatric or neurological diseases, side effects of medications or social deprivation. Very few studies have addressed the diagnosis and treatment of secondary negative symptoms (Kirschner, Aleman, and Kaiser, 2017). Box.1.1 includes a case vignette of a hypothetical patients with secondary negative symptoms.

1.3.1.1 Negative symptoms secondary to positive symptoms

In most cases there is no need for specific interventions in addition to antipsychotic treatment for positive symptoms. If the negative symptoms emerged or (if they were already present before the positive symptoms started or increased) increased due to positive symptoms, the improvement of positive symptoms is expected to be associated with the improvement of the negative symptoms.

However, high doses of antipsychotics for the treatment of positive symptoms may cause increased severity of negative symptoms, by potentially causing extrapyramidal symptoms, anhedonia, depression, and sedation. The lowering of the plasma levels of haloperidol after the first three weeks of acute treatment below

---

Box 1.1

The differential diagnosis of primary versus secondary negative symptoms may be very difficult. For example:

1. At admission to a psychiatric unit, a patient with an acute episode of schizophrenia has predominant positive symptoms and an increased level of negative symptoms as compared to their level before the onset of the acute episode—the increase in negative symptoms maybe *secondary to positive symptoms*.

2. Antipsychotic treatment was started. The severity of positive symptoms decreased, however the patient developed mild hypokinesia, and the level of negative symptoms increased further. This increase may be considered as *secondary to extrapyramidal symptoms*.

3. The severity of positive symptoms continued to decrease, however the patient developed a major depressive episode, and the severity of negative symptoms increased further, which may be considered as *secondary to depressive symptoms*. A mildly fluctuating but continuing decrease in the severity of positive symptoms resulted in predominantly negative symptoms, since the level of the severity of negative symptoms exceeded the severity of positive symptoms. The dose of antipsychotic was decreased and the patient received an antiparkinsonian drug for a few days—the severity of negative symptoms started decreasing. After two weeks hypokinesia was no longer detectable, however the patient remained depressed. Depression improved slowly without antidepressant treatment and the negative symptoms improved parallel to the improvement of depression. This improvement might have been the result of improvement in *negative symptoms secondary to depression*. Twelve months later the patient had mild positive symptoms with persistent, predominant negative symptoms and no depressive or extrapyramidal symptoms; at this point the patient fulfilled the criteria for deficit schizophrenia.

---

12 ng/ml (current recommendations: 1–10 ng/ml; alert level: 15 ng/ml; (Hiemke, Bergemann, Clement, et al. 2018) reduced negative symptoms (Volavka, Cooper, Czobor, et al. 1995).

1.3.1.2 Negative symptoms secondary to EPS

EPS side effects of antipsychotic treatment (mainly hypokinesia) are underdiagnosed. The recognition and differential diagnosis of mild hypokinesia requires special attention and training. Handwriting samples may reveal micrographia, which is associated with hypokinesia during antipsychotic treatment (Bitter, Volavka, and Scheurer, 1991). If EPS persist, a decrease of the dose of or change in antipsychotic medication should be considered. Treatment with antiparkinsonian drugs can be recommended but only for a short time: dopaminergic antiparkinsonian drugs are contraindicated in schizophrenia since they can exacerbate positive symptoms, and anticholinergic drugs have many side effects, including cognitive disturbances and sedation, which may contribute to the increase of the severity of secondary negative symptoms.

1.3.1.3 Negative symptoms secondary to depression

Depression is a frequent symptom in the course of schizophrenia and 'full-blown' major depressive episodes are estimated to affect one-third of the patients with the diagnosis of schizophrenia, and another one-third may have fluctuating symptoms of depression; first episode/younger patients seem to be at higher risk for this comorbidity (Dai, Du, Yin, et al. 2018). The use of depression rating scales can be recommended for severity assessment. The Calgary Depression Rating Scale (CDRS) (Addington, Addington, and Maticka-Tyndale, 1993), which was specifically designed for the measurement of depression in schizophrenia, may have some advantages, however other scales are also useful.

1.3.1.4 Negative symptoms secondary to substance use

About half of the patients with schizophrenia are affected by substance-related disorders in their life. Substance abuse increases morbidity and mortality and contributes to the increase of both positive and negative symptoms in schizophrenia (Volkow, 2009). Unfortunately, depression and EPS may also be comorbid in this group of patients. Chronic use, intoxication, and withdrawal may all contribute to negative symptoms. The treatment of patients with the dual diagnosis of schizophrenia and substance use-related disorders is one of the most difficult tasks in psychiatry.

1.3.1.5 Negative symptoms secondary to other neurological or psychiatric disorders

This group of disorders/diseases is important for the differential diagnosis of schizophrenia and/or as comorbid conditions of schizophrenia as well. The list is a reminder, rather than standing as a complete list of potential conditions: anxiety/anxiety disorders, mental retardation, extrapyramidal diseases (e.g. Parkinson's disease, Wilson's disease), tumours of the central nervous system, Alzheimer disease and other dementias, encephalitis (especially difficult to diagnose autoimmune encephalitis, e.g. anti-NMDA (N-methyl-D-aspartate) receptor encephalitis), Lyme disease.

1.3.1.6 Negative symptoms secondary to social deprivation and other social disadvantages

The psychological consequences of deprivation and isolation—especially in the childhood—include negative symptoms, such as emotional withdrawal or anhedonia.

Hospitalizations became shorter worldwide in the last decades, however recent research supports the contribution of the disease ('persistence of the poor outcome processes' of schizophrenia) to extended institutional stay rather than the contribution of hospital treatment to poor outcomes (e.g. Harvey, Loewenstein, and Czaja, 2013).

Further research in schizophrenia is needed on how to interpret recent data about the effects of low income and major financial loss ('negative wealth shock'), which has been found to be associated with excess mortality as compared to higher income groups and to people with positive wealth without negative wealth shock (Chetty, Stepner, Abraham, et al. 2016; Pool, Burgard, Needham, et al. 2018).

The evaluation of negative symptoms has to consider the options available to patients. People with the diagnosis of schizophrenia are often financially disadvantaged and have no access to those activities which are often used in the measurement of negative symptoms.

1.3.2 Type I and Type II schizophrenia

Crow (1980) emphasized the potential existence of two 'disease processes': Type I schizophrenia has positive symptoms associated with relatively good premorbid adjustment, good responsiveness to 'traditional' antipsychotics, and fair outcome. Type II schizophrenia is characterized by negative symptoms associated with relatively poor premorbid adjustment, poor responsiveness to 'traditional' antipsychotics, and poor outcome. Crow hypothesized that Type I schizophrenia is associated with abnormal neurotransmitter activity and Type II schizophrenia with abnormal brain structures.

1.3.3 Persistent negative symptoms (PNS)

As mentioned earlier, the persistence of negative symptoms defines a specific group and the term *persistent primary negative symptoms* defines an even smaller group by excluding patients with enduring secondary negative symptoms.

PNS has been defined as negative symptoms of at least moderate severity for an extended period of time (usually 6 or 12 months) in the presence of low levels of positive, depressive, and extrapyramidal symptoms; the evaluation of PNS requires evaluation with rating scales (Buchanan, 2007).

1.3.4 Prominent negative symptoms

Prominent negative symptoms (and prominent positive symptoms) were defined as baseline score ≥ 4 (moderate) on at least three, or ≥ 5 (moderately severe) on at least two negative (or positive) PANSS subscale items (Rabinowitz, Berardo, Bugarski-Kirola, et al. 2013). When persistent primary negative symptoms are present for a long period of time then prominent positive symptoms during an acute episode do not invalidate their diagnosis.

1.3.5 Predominant negative symptoms

There are a few definitions of predominant negative symptoms with different criteria, for example a PANSS negative subscale score of at least 21 and at least 1 point greater than the PANSS positive subscale, or the PANSS negative subscale score at least 6 points higher than the PANSS positive subscale score. A simple definition is probably the most frequently used: the PANSS negative subscale score is greater than the positive one (Rabinowitz, et al. 2013).

The EMA guideline 'Clinical investigation of medicinal products, including depot preparations in the treatment of schizophrenia' includes a chapter on efficacy on negative symptoms which states: 'If an effect on negative symptoms is claimed, specially designed studies in patients with predominant negative symptoms should be conducted' (EMA, 2012).

The usefulness of inclusion of the term 'predominant' in the EMA guidelines is at the very least controversial (e.g. Mucci, Merlotti, Üçok, et al. 2017). Positive and negative symptoms are in many patients 'desynchronized': negative symptoms often start earlier than the onset of positive symptoms and positive symptoms may have a relapsing–remitting/partially remitting course, while negative symptoms usually follow a slightly fluctuating course and their severity may increase over time. The increases in the severity of negative symptoms may be associated with increases in severity of positive symptoms (relapses or acute episodes), however in a significant proportion of patients negative symptoms do not improve or improve rather less than positive symptoms do during treatment of an acute episode (relapse). The course of schizophrenia may include periods with predominant positive symptoms during relapses and periods with predominant negative symptoms between relapses. If the period between two relapses is characterized by predominant negative symptoms and this period lasts more than six months, then the criteria for predominant and persistent negative symptoms are met; during the next relapse with predominant positive symptoms and even with the same or even increased severity of persistent negative symptoms the criteria for 'predominant and persistent negative symptoms' will no longer be met. It is important to note that negative symptoms may be difficult to evaluate during relapses with acute positive symptoms. Thus 'persistent negative symptoms' or 'persistent primary negative symptoms' would be the preferable terms for capturing enduring primary negative symptoms as treatment targets. The definitions 'predominant negative symptoms' and 'prominent negative symptoms' remain controversial; they exclude a significant number of patients with persistent primary negative symptoms from clinical studies and may negatively impact their access to treatment.

Fig. 1.1 presents the complexity of primary versus secondary negative symptoms and of predominant positive versus predominant negative symptoms.

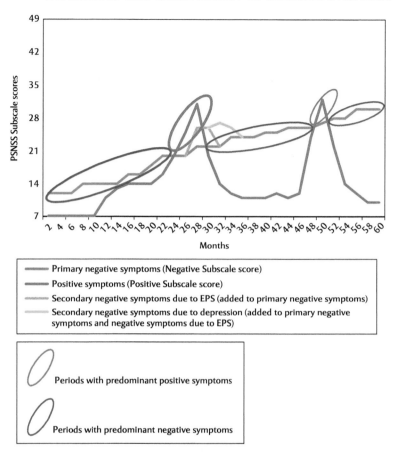

Figure 1.1 Course of positive and primary and secondary negative symptoms in a period of 60 months, including the first and second episodes of schizophrenia (in a hypothetical patient).

1.4 Deficit schizophrenia

The definition of deficit schizophrenia requires the presence of persistent primary negative symptoms; the criteria are summarized in Box 1.2 (Kirkpatrick, Buchanan, McKenny, et al. 1989).

Box 1.2 Diagnostic criteria for the deficit syndrome of schizophrenia

1. At least two of the following six negative symptoms must be present:
   a. Restricted affect
   b. Diminished emotional range
   c. Poverty of speech
   d. Curbing of interests
   e. Diminished sense of purpose
   f. Diminished social drive
2. Some combination of two or more of the negative symptoms listed above have been present for the preceding 12 months and were always present during periods of clinical stability (including chronic psychotic states). These symptoms may or may not be detectable during transient episodes of acute psychotic disorganization or decompensation.
3. The negative symptoms above are primary, that is, not secondary to factors of another disease process. Such factors include:
   a. anxiety
   b. drug effect
   c. suspiciousness (and other psychotic symptoms)
   d. mental retardation
   e. depression
4. The patient meets DSM criteria for schizophrenia.

Reproduced courtesy of Dr Brian Kirkpatrick.

1.5 Rating scales for the measurement of negative symptoms

The aims of this chapter include to provide the readers with practical information on rating scales for the evaluation of negative symptoms in schizophrenia, however a comprehensive review of the available negative symptom scales or even a listing of all negative symptom scales is beyond the scope of this book. The inclusion of some scales in the Appendix of the book in addition to two other chapters of this book addressing the measurement of negative symptoms (Chapter 2 on basic symptoms; Chapter 4 on self-evaluation of negative symptoms) helps the readers gain a better insight into the variety of negative symptoms and the variability of their definitions.

The EMA guidelines discussed in box 1.3 (EMA, 2012) recommend for clinical trials that 'improvement on negative symptoms should be demonstrated through validated scales (e.g. PANSS negative subscale, SANS or other), and presented as the difference between baseline and endpoint. Responder rates should be provided and demonstration of functional improvement, e.g. improvement in functional capacity, as key secondary outcome measure is recommended.'

Box 1.3 EMA guidelines

The EMA guideline lists the following criteria 'to ensure that patients with true negative symptoms of schizophrenia are studied':

'Inclusion criteria should encompass:

a) Predominant and persistent negative symptoms.
b) Flat affect, poverty of speech, and avolition being present as representative of core negative symptoms.
c) Stable condition of schizophrenic illness for longer than 6 months, especially of the negative symptoms.

Exclusion criteria should include:

d) Major depression; low depression scores are preferable.
e) Subjects with substantially confounding extra-pyramidal symptoms.
f) Substantial non-compliance or substance abuse.'

In a recent review, the authors concluded that 'a) the assessment of the negative symptom dimension has recently improved, but even current expert consensus-based instruments diverge on several aspects; b) the use of objective measures might contribute to overcome uncertainties about the reliability of rating scales, but these measures require further investigation and validation' (Marder and Galderisi, 2017).

The NIMH-MATRICS consensus statement on negative symptoms (Kirkpatrick, et al. 2006) acknowledged that PANSS and SANS and other instruments are appropriate for use in clinical trials, and it also stated that the structure of SANS is preferable to that of the PANSS.

The Brief Psychiatric Rating Scale (BPRS) is 'the classic' in the group (Overall and Gorham, 1962) and has a well-documented negative factor consisting of three items: blunted affect, emotional withdrawal, and motor retardation. When using only a single factor score for characterizing negative symptoms, the BPRS negative factor is still a valuable measurement tool (Czobor, Bitter, and Volavka, 1991).

The PANSS includes seven items in its negative subscale (Kay, Fiszbein, and Opler, 1987), however a number of factor analytic studies of PANSS suggested other items as negative than only those originally included in its negative subscale. Table 1.1 compares the negative symptoms included in the negative subscale of PANSS with the symptoms included in the negative factor suggested by Marder and colleagues (1997). The original negative subscale of PANSS and their modified versions (negative factors of the PANSS) are frequently used in clinical trials.

The SANS (Andreasen, 1982) consists of five negative symptom domains (affective flattening or blunting, alogia, avolition–apathy, anhedonia–asociality, and attention). Each domain covers two to six symptoms and has a global rating. The scale has been frequently used for measuring changes during clinical trials.

Table 1.1 The comparison of negative symptoms in the negative subscale of PANSS and a negative factor of PANSS

PANSS Negative	Subscale (Kay, et al. 1987)	Factor (Marder, et al. 1997)
Blunted affect	+	+
Emotional withdrawal	+	+
Poor rapport	+	+
Passive/apathetic social withdrawal	+	+
Difficulty in abstract thinking	+	-
Lack of spontaneity and flow of conversation	+	+
Stereotyped thinking	+	-
Motor retardation	-	+
Active social avoidance	-	+

Source data from: Kay, S. R., Fiszbein, A., Opler, L. A. (1987). The positive and negative syndrome scale (PANSS) for schizophrenia. *Schizophrenia Bulletin*, 13, pp. 261–76; Marder, S. R., Davis, J. M., Chouinard, G. (1997). The effects of risperidone on the five dimensions of schizophrenia derived by factor analysis: combined results of the North American trials. *Journal of Clinical Psychiatry*, 58, pp. 538–46.

The SANS is included in the Appendix of this book with the kind permission of Dr Andreasen. The definitions of the individual symptoms/items of SANS summarize the characteristics of the negative syndrome in schizophrenia.

The Negative Symptom Assessment (NSA) (Alphs, Summerfelt, Lann, et al. 1989) is also a frequently used instrument. It consisted originally of 25 items, which was shortened to 16 items (NSA-16). NSA-16 is best described by five factors (Communication, Social Involvement, Affect/Emotion, Motivation, and Retardation) (Axelrod, Goldman, and Alphs, 1993). A short version consisting of four items (NSA-4) was also developed and it demonstrated that NSA-4 offers accuracy comparable to the NSA-16 in rating negative symptoms in patients with schizophrenia (Alphs, Morlock, Coon, et al. 2011). The NSA-16 and NSA-4 are included in the Appendix of this book with the kind permission of Dr Alphs.

The Brief Negative Symptom Scale (BNSS) is a more recently introduced rating scale consisting of 13 items. It covers the five domains recommended by the NIMH-MATRICS consensus statement on negative symptoms: blunted affect, alogia, asociality, anhedonia, and avolition. It includes an item on the self-reported lack of normal distress, which is a frequently observed symptom in patients with negative symptoms. The scale has been translated in a number of languages (Bischof, Obermann, Hartmann, et al. 2016; Mucci, Vignapiano, Bitter, et al. 2019) and has been used both in Europe and in the United States in clinical trials evaluating change in negative symptoms. A table listing the items of BNSS and example probes for some of the items are included with in the Appendix the kind permission of Dr Kirkpatrick and Dr Strauss, and of ProPhase LLC.

Recent data suggest that negative symptoms are best conceptualized in relation to the five consensus domains (Strauss, Nuñez, Ahmed, et al. 2018), and the five-factor structure of negative symptoms in schizophrenia was successfully confirmed in the process of cross-cultural validation (Ahmed, Kirkpatrick, Galderisi, et al. 2018).

Using the total scores of sophisticated rating scales as a single numerical measure of the presence and severity of negative symptoms unfortunately does not reflect the wealth of information included in the individual items of the respective scales. Aggregating the ratings of individual items into one factor score results in the loss of information. The use of two or more scales for the measurement of negative symptoms results in various levels of redundancy; factor analytic studies present the variables that are most effective in describing variance, however we should consider that they can also be highly redundant. In one of our earlier works addressing this important topic we came to the following conclusion: 'the elimination of the overlapping variance … is not only a statistical problem: the lack of redundancy in a statistical sense does not necessarily mean useful psychometric information. Yet, adequate knowledge of a scale's interset relationship is indispensable for further research. As the number of standardized scales increases, psychometric research should incorporate information about their interset relationships' (Czobor, et al. 1991).

1.5 Conclusion

Recent research data and input from regulatory agencies (EMA, FDA) helped in the reconceptualization of negative symptoms. Current evidence supports five factors, the five 'As' of negative symptoms: blunted affect, alogia, asociality, anhedonia, and avolition. Persistent primary negative symptoms emerged as targets for new treatments; the regulatory guidance of selecting patients with *predominant* negative symptoms for clinical trials has not been supported by research evidence. According to the NIMH-MATRIX expert consensus, the PANSS, SANS, and other assessment approaches are appropriate for application in current clinical trials. The Negative Symptom Assessment (NSA) has a short, four-item version. The recently developed Brief Negative Symptom Scale (BNSS) covers the five factors described earlier with good validity and reliability.

Further research is needed about the relationships of various negative symptom scales and about the usefulness of the inclusion/exclusion of specific items into those scales for the clinical practice and research.

REFERENCES

Addington, D., Addington,J., Maticka-Tyndale, E. (1993). Assessing depression in schizophrenia: the Calgary Depression Scale. *British Journal of Psychiatry*, **163**(S22), 39–44.

Ahmed, A. O., Kirkpatrick, B., Galderisi, S., Mucci, A., Rossi, A., Bertolino, A., et al. (2018). Cross-cultural validation of the 5-factor structure of negative symptoms in schizophrenia. *Schizophrenia Bulletin*, **45**(2), 305–14.

Alphs, L. D., Summerfelt, A., Lann, H., Muller, R. J. (1989). The Negative Symptom Assessment: a new instrument to assess negative symptoms in schizophrenia. *Psychopharmacology Bulletin*, **25**, 159–63.

Alphs, L., Morlock, R., Coon, C., Cazorla, P., Szegedi, A., Panagides, J. (2011). Validation of a 4-item Negative Symptom Assessment (NSA-4): a short, practical clinical tool for the assessment of negative symptoms in schizophrenia. *International Journal of Methods in Psychiatric Research*, **20**(2), e31–e37.

Andreasen, N. C. (1982). Negative symptoms in schizophrenia: definition and reliability. *Archives of General Psychiatry*, **39**(7), 784–8.

Axelrod, B. N., Goldman, R. S., Alphs, L. D. (1993). Validation of the 16-item negative symptom assessment. *Journal of Psychiatric Research*, **27**(3), 253–8.

Bischof, M., Obermann, C., Hartmann, M. N., Hager, O. M., Kirschner, M., Kluge, A., et al. (2016). The brief negative symptom scale: validation of the German translation and convergent validity with self-rated anhedonia and observer-rated apathy. *BMC Psychiatry*, **16**(1), 415.

Bitter, I., Jaeger, J., Agdeppa, J., Volavka, J. (1989). Subjective symptoms: part of the negative syndrome of schizophrenia? *Psychopharmacology Bulletin*, **25**(2), 180–4.

Bitter, I., Volavka, J., Scheurer, J. (1991). The concept of the neuroleptic threshold: an update. *Journal of Clinical Psychopharmacology*, **11**(1), 28–33.

Bleuler, E. (1983). *Lehrbuch der Psychiatrie. 15. Auflage, neubearbeitet von Manfred Bleuler.* New York, Springer.

Buchanan, R. W. (2007). Persistent negative symptoms in schizophrenia: an overview. *Schizophrenia Bulletin*, **33**(4), 1013–22.

Chetty, R., Stepner, M., Abraham, S., Lin, S., Scuderi, B., Turner, N., et al. (2016). The association between income and life expectancy in the United States, 2001–2014. *Journal of the American Medical Association*, **315**(16), 1750–66.

Crow, T. J. (1980). Molecular pathology of schizophrenia: more than one disease process? *British Medical Journal*, **280**(6207), 66.

Czobor, P., Bitter, I., Volavka, J. (1991). Relationship between the Brief Psychiatric Rating Scale and the Scale for the Assessment of Negative Symptoms: a study of their correlation and redundancy. *Psychiatry Research*, **36**(2), 129–39.

Dai, J., Du, X., Yin, G., Zhang, Y., Xia, H., Li, X., et al. (2018). Prevalence, demographic and clinical features of comorbid depressive symptoms in drug naive patients with schizophrenia presenting with first episode psychosis. *Schizophrenia Research*, **193**, 182–7.

EMA (2012). Clinical investigation of medicinal products, including depot preparations in the treatment of schizophrenia. (Effective from 1 April 2013). https://www.ema. europa.eu/en/clinical-investigation-medicinal-products-including-depot-preparations-treatment-schizophrenia. Last accessed: 24 May 2019.

Galderisi, S., Mucci, A., Bitter, I., Libiger, J., Bucci, P., Fleischhacker, W.W., et al. (2013). Persistent negative symptoms in first episode patients with schizophrenia: results from the European First Episode Schizophrenia Trial. *European Neuropsychopharmacology*, **22**, 196–204.

Gard, D. E., Kring, A. M., Gard, M. G., Horan, W. P., Green, M. F. (2007). Anhedonia in schizophrenia: distinctions between anticipatory and consummatory pleasure. *Schizophrenia Research*, **93**(1–3), 253–60.

Harvey, P. D., Loewenstein, D. A., Czaja, S. J. (2013). Hospitalization and psychosis: influences on the course of cognition and everyday functioning in people with schizophrenia. *Neurobiology of Disease*, **53**, 18–25.

Hiemke, C., Bergemann, N., Clement, H. W., Conca, A., Deckert, J., Domschke, K., et al. (2018). Consensus guidelines for therapeutic drug monitoring in neuropsychopharmacology: update 2017. *Pharmacopsychiatry*, **51**(01/02), 9–62.

Horan, W. P., Kring, A. M., Gur, R. E., Reise, S.P., Blanchard, J. J. (2011). Development and psychometric validation of the Clinical Assessment Interview for Negative Symptoms (CAINS). Schizophrenia Research, **132**, 140–5.

Jackson, J. H. (1887). Remarks on evolution and dissolution of the nervous system. *Journal of Mental Science*, **33**, 25–48.

Kay, S. R., Fiszbein, A., Opler, L. A. (1987). The Positive and Negative Syndrome Scale (PANSS) for schizophrenia. *Schizophrenia Bulletin*, **13**, 261–76.

Kirkpatrick, B., Buchanan, R. W., McKenny, P. D., Alphs, L. D., Carpenter Jr, W. T. (1989). The schedule for the deficit syndrome: an instrument for research in schizophrenia. *Psychiatry Research*, **30**(2), 119–23.

Kirkpatrick, B., Fenton, W. S., Carpenter, W. T., Marder, S. R. (2006). The NIMH-MATRICS consensus statement on negative symptoms. *Schizophrenia Bulletin*, **32**(2), 214–19.

Kirschner, M., Aleman, A., Kaiser, S. (2017). Secondary negative symptoms—a review of mechanisms, assessment and treatment. *Schizophrenia Research*, **186**, 29–38.

Komlósi, S., Csukly, G., Stefanics, G., Czigler, I., Bitter, I., Czobor, P. (2013). Fearful face recognition in schizophrenia: An electrophysiological study. *Schizophrenia Research*, **149**(1–3), 135–40.

Kraepelin, E. (1904). *Psychiatrie. Ein Lehrbuch für Studierende und Ärzte. Siebente, vielfach überarbeitete Auflage. II. Band. Klinische Psychiatrie.* Leipzig, Verlag von Johann Ambrosius Barth.

Laughren, T., Levin, R. (2006). Food and Drug Administration perspective on negative symptoms in schizophrenia as a target for a drug treatment claim. *Schizophrenia Bulletin*, **32**, 220–2.

Marder, S. R., Davis, J. M., Chouinard, G. (1997). The effects of risperidone on the five dimensions of schizophrenia derived by factor analysis: combined results of the North American trials. *Journal of Clinical Psychiatry*, **58**, 538–46.

Marder, S. R., Galderisi, S. (2017). The current conceptualization of negative symptoms in schizophrenia. *World Psychiatry*, **16**(1), 14–24.

Mucci, A., Merlotti, E., Üçok, A., Aleman, A., Galderisi, S. (2017). Primary and persistent negative symptoms: concepts, assessments and neurobiological bases. *Schizophrenia Research*, **186**, 19–28.

Mucci, A., Vignapiano, A., Bitter, I., Austin, S. F., Delouche, C., Dollfus, S., et al. (2019). A large European, multicenter, multinational validation study of the Brief Negative Symptom Scale. *European Neuropsychopharmacology*. In press

Overall, J. E., Gorham, D. R. (1962). The Brief Psychiatric Rating Scale. *Psychological Reports*, **10**, 799–812.

Pool, L. R., Burgard, S. A., Needham, B. L., Elliott, M. R., Langa, K. M., De Leon, C. F. M. (2018). Association of a negative wealth shock with all-cause mortality in middle-aged and older adults in the United States. *Journal of the American Medical Association*, **319**(13), 1341–50.

Rabinowitz, J., Berardo, C. G., Bugarski-Kirola, D., Marder, S. (2013). Association of prominent positive and prominent negative symptoms and functional health, well-being, healthcare-related quality of life and family burden: a CATIE analysis. *Schizophrenia Research*, **150**(2–3), 339–42.

Schneider, K. (1980). *Klinische Psychopathologie*. 12. Auflage. Stuttgart, Georg Thieme Verlag.

Strauss, G. P., Nuñez, A., Ahmed, A. O., Barchard, K. A., Granholm, E., Kirkpatrick, B., et al. (2018). The latent structure of negative symptoms in schizophrenia. *Journal of the American Medical Association Psychiatry*, **75**(12), 1271–1279.

Volavka, J., Cooper, T. B., Czobor, P., Meisner, M. (1995). Plasma Haloperidol Levels and Clinical Effects in Schizophrenia and Schizoaffective Disorder. *Archives of General Psychiatry*, **52**(10), 837–45.

Volkow, N. D. (2009). Substance use disorders in schizophrenia—clinical implications of comorbidity. *Schizophrenia Bulletin*, **35**(3), 469–72.

CHAPTER 2

Basic symptoms in deficit states and their relation to negative symptoms

Frauke Schultze-Lutter

KEY POINTS

* Basic symptoms are subtle, subjectively experienced disturbances in mental processes including thinking, speech, attention, perception, drive, stress tolerance, and affect, originally described by Gerd Huber.

* Basic symptoms are present in prodromal, psychotic, and residual/deficit states of schizophrenia and have been conceptualized as the most immediate psychopathological expression of the neurobiological abnormalities underlying the development and persistence of psychosis.

* Basic symptoms are currently mostly recognized for their potential to detect psychosis prior to the first psychotic episode and, thus, for their ability to herald persistent positive symptoms.

* Although initially described to facilitate understanding of deficit states in schizophrenia, their contribution to negative symptoms has been less studied, although the evaluation of basic symptoms helps in improving understanding of the psychopathology—including differentiation of primary and secondary negative symptoms—and course of schizophrenia and in planning better treatment.

Knowledge of basic symptoms and of the stages and modalities of their development can be used in research and the clinic, for diagnostic and differential-diagnostic purposes, for therapy and rehabilitation, and in particular for the early detection, early intervention and (secondary) prevention of psychosis.

2.1 The basic symptom concept

Tracing back to early descriptions of prodromal symptoms of Wilhelm Mayer-Gross (1932), the concept of basic symptoms (BS) was gradually developed by

Gerd Huber in the 1960s (Huber, 1995; 1996), who was also the first to describe enlarged ventricles *in vivo* in patients with schizophrenia (Huber, 1996). Against the background of his pneumoencephalographic research, Huber chose the term *basic* symptoms for their assumed 'substrate closeness', that is his perception of BS as the earliest primarily subjective psychopathological correlates of the neurobiological disturbances of information processing underlying the development of psychosis (Huber, 1966; Schultze-Lutter, 2009; Schultze-Lutter, Ruhrmann, Fusar-Poli, et al. 2012b; Schultze-Lutter, Debbané, Theodoridou, et al. 2016; Schultze-Lutter, Ruhrmann, Kindler, et al. 2018b). BS have thus been considered as an integral part of psychosis and to appear throughout all stages of the disorder (Schultze-Lutter, 2009; Schultze-Lutter, et al. 2012b; Schultze-Lutter and Theodoridou, 2017), although they are not per se specific to psychosis and might occur in other severe non-organic mental disorders, in particular affective disorders (Klosterkötter, Ebel, Schultze-Lutter, et al. 1996).

BS are subtle, subclinical disturbances in all dimensions of mental processes such as drive, affect, stress tolerance, thinking, speech, sensory perception, body perception, motor action and central-vegetative functions that are self-experienced with immediate and full insight into their abnormal nature (Gross and Huber, 1989; Schultze-Lutter, 2009; Schultze-Lutter, et al. 2012b). Consequently, the ability to experience BS with insight and to report them often weakens with progressive illness, i.e., with loss of insight and emerging positive psychotic symptoms, but is commonly restored upon remission (Gross and Huber, 1989). For their self-experienced deviation from the normal self, a subgroup of BS—only three of them relating to drive and affect—in combination with selected attenuated psychotic symptoms and related symptoms have later been conceptualized as 'self-disturbances' or self-disorders and a core schizophrenia vulnerability phenotype (Parnas, Møller, Kircher, et al. 2005).

The original BS concept distinguished between three permeable symptom dimensions—or stages—of different severity and specificity to psychoses (Gross and Huber, 1989; Schultze-Lutter, 2009; Schultze-Lutter, et al. 2016). Upon debut at stage 1, first unspecific BS will occur, which mainly involve disturbances of drive, volition, affect, concentration, attention, and memory that phenomenologically resemble negative symptoms. However, they may be distinguishable from negative symptoms in their current understanding in that they are not necessarily observable functional deficits (Marder and Galderisi, 2017) but predominately private. At stage 2, these unspecific BS will be followed by the occurrence of qualitatively peculiar and presumably more specific BS, including disturbances of thinking, speech, sensory perception, body perception, and motor action, which will gradually increase in number and severity. In most cases and based on BS, attenuated and frank positive psychotic symptoms will ultimately develop at stage 3, although temporary improvements are possible (Huber, 1986; Gross and Huber, 1989; Schultze-Lutter, 2009; Schultze-Lutter, et al. 2016). In some cases, BS will even spontaneously remit completely before reoccurring and developing into full-blown psychotic symptoms. Because these symptomatic phases, which can mimic true prodromal stages, potentially announce the subsequent prodrome, they were called *outpost syndromes* (Gross and Huber, 1989; Schultze-Lutter, 2009).

Furthermore, the BS concept assumes that, following the first episode of psychosis, BS will evolve into one of three different types of outcome (Gross and Huber, 1989). One is a good outcome with persistent full remission of BS and other symptoms; the second is a partially poor outcome with only temporary full or partial remission and relapse episodes; and the third is a poor outcome with persistence of BS, especially of disturbances in drive, stress tolerance, affect, i.e., BS resembling negative symptoms, and cognition (Gross and Huber, 1989). The role of these symptoms in predicting relapse was recently supported (Gaebel and Riesbeck, 2014; Eisner, Drake, Lobban, et al. 2018), whereby a huge neglect of BS by clinicians became obvious (Eisner, et al. 2018). However, studies of BS in the manifest psychosis and its course are only just emerging; the majority of studies in the past 30 years focused on the role of BS in the prediction of psychosis (Schultze-Lutter and Theodoridou, 2017).

2.2 Development of negative, disorganized, and positive symptoms from basic symptoms

The BS model of the development of psychoses assumes that neurobiological aberrations impair information processing at a cerebral level (Schultze-Lutter, et al. 2016; 2018b). The resulting pathologically vulnerable information processing capacity then becomes more susceptible to negative effects of stress. Consequently, already everyday situations and demands will more quickly overstrain the remaining information processing capacity and trigger the development of first stage-1 and later of characteristic stage-2 BS and their conversion to (attenuated) positive, and other disorganized, and primary and secondary negative symptoms (Gross and Huber, 1989; Schultze-Lutter, 2009; Schultze-Lutter, et al. 2016;). Yet, if environmental and personal conditions are favourable (e.g., if there is a supportive social network, and the person possesses good social, problem solving and coping skills), BS can well be coped with at any state as long as their number and/or severity do not overstrain personal resources. For this reason, in early phases, the emerging disorder will only become apparent to others, when inadequate coping strategies are employed or when compensatory abilities are exhausted and, consequently, BS start to interfere with behaviour. Thus, others might observe patients' self-initiated coping strategies (avoidance strategies, compensatory behaviors and/or self-medication) and emotional reactions (such as feelings of helplessness, anxiety, tension and/or confusion) in response to BS, e.g., as primary or secondary negative, or affective symptoms, or suicidality (Schmidt, Schultze-Lutter, Bendall, et al. 2017). That is to say, BS of any kind might become apparent as functional deficits or negative symptoms (e.g., avolition, attentional impairment, alogia, anhedonia incl. asociality, and affective flattening), as disorganized communication and behaviour, and/or as other changes in affect and emotional stability. For example, social withdrawal presenting as asociality and/or avolition might directly result from a significantly decreased ability to tolerate social interactions, or from a loss of energy or of drive, or might simply be a result of a decrease in the wish for social contacts that is acted upon. Yet, asociality in terms of a secondary negative symptom might as well result from inadequate coping with disturbances of receptive or expressive speech, or a decrease in thought initiative (that might result in feeling incompetent in social communication and, consequently, in avoiding them). Alternatively, or in addition, disturbances of receptive and expressive speech or a decrease in thought initiative as well as other cognitive disturbances, when severe and frequent, might as well become observable as primary attentional impairment.

On the other hand, BS might become observable by others when insight cannot be maintained and inadequate explanatory models are developed that might present as attenuated or frank delusional or hallucinatory psychotic symptoms (Gross and Huber, 1989; Schultze-Lutter, 2009; Schultze-Lutter, et al. 2018b). The assumption that BS primarily relate to neurobiological correlates and brain maturation, and (attenuated) positive symptoms primarily to neuropsychological correlates and maturation of cognitive abilities was recently supported by age effects on the prevalence and clinical significance of BS and attenuated positive symptoms in the 8- to 40-year-old general population (Schimmelmann, Michel, Martz-Irngartinger, et al. 2015; Schultze-Lutter, et al. 2018b).

2.3 Basic symptoms in the prediction of psychosis

Cross-sectional studies indicated that the majority of BS—in particular those phenomenologically resembling negative symptoms as well as body perception disturbances—are not specific to psychosis and may occur in other, especially non-psychotic affective disorders (Klosterkötter, Ebel, Schultze-Lutter, et al. 1996; Klosterkötter, Gross, Huber, et al. 1997; Schultze-Lutter, et al. 2012b). Yet, the first long-term prospective early detection study (Klosterkötter, Hellmich, Steinmeyer, et al. 2001) found that altogether 14 cognitive and perceptive BS (see Box 2.1) were specific to the development of first-episode schizophrenia. These were employed in two partially overlapping BS criteria (see Box 2.1), Cognitive-Perceptive Basic Symptoms (COPER) and Cognitive Disturbances (COGDIS) (Klosterkötter, et al. 2001; Schultze-Lutter, Ruhrmann, and Klosterkötter, 2006; Schultze-Lutter, Klosterkötter, Picker, et al. 2007b).

COGDIS, in particular, was related to conversion rates at least as high as those reported for the ultra-high risk (UHR) criteria (Yung, Phillips, McGorry, et al. 1998) in a recent meta-analysis and, thus, recommended for the diagnosis of a psychosis-risk state within the framework of the guidance project of the European Psychiatric Association (Schultze-Lutter, Michel, Schmidt, et al. 2015). Furthermore, an earlier meta-analysis on the type of psychosis upon conversion in psychosis-risk samples had linked BS criteria to a higher likelihood of developing schizophrenia—and, thereby, of developing severe negative

Box 2.1 Basic symptom criteria and definitions of relevant symptoms

COGNITIVE DISTURBANCES (COGDIS)

At least any two of the following nine basic symptoms with a SPI-A or SPI-CY score of at least '3' (i.e. at least weekly occurrence) within the last three months:

Inability to divide attention: A difficulty in dealing with demands—commonly one being a task requiring very little attention—that involve more than one sensory modality at a time and, thus, does not concern demands that would require quick switching of attention. This BS might be the subjective counterpart of *attentional impairment* or *avolition* as a primary negative symptom.

Captivation of attention by details of the visual field: Domination of the visual field by a random single aspect that captures the person's whole attention, impedes attention to other aspects, and causes difficulties in turning away from it. This BS might be the subjective counterpart of *attentional impairment* as a primary negative symptom.

Thought interference: Insignificant thoughts, which are unrelated to the intended thought, intrude and disturb the person's train of thought, without the intended thought getting lost. This BS might be the subjective counterpart of *attentional impairment* as a primary negative symptom.

Thought pressure: A self-reported 'chaos' of thoughts in which successively occurring thoughts are not linked by any common thread, are completely unrelated to each other, and to the person's intended line of thought. This BS might be the subjective counterpart of *attentional impairment* as a primary negative symptom.

Thought blockages: Sudden interruption in the flow of thoughts, experiences of the mind suddenly or gradually going blank, or losing the thread of thoughts. The original topic is either lost completely or subsequently recalled. This BS might be the subjective counterpart of *attentional impairment* and/or *alogia* as a primary negative symptom and/or *anhedonia* (*asociality*) as a secondary negative symptom, if leading to avoid conversations, that is, to social withdrawal.

Disturbance of receptive speech: A disturbance in the understanding of simple everyday words. When reading or listening to others, the person struggles to comprehend the meaning of words, word sequences, or sentences, even if the person concentrates on the text or speech. This BS might be the subjective counterpart of *attentional impairment* as a primary negative symptom and/or *anhedonia* (*asociality*) as a secondary negative symptom, if leading to avoid conversations, that is, to social withdrawal.

Disturbance of expressive speech: A subjective difficulty in verbal fluency and clarity of expression, with words required to express simple ideas being not forthcoming or delayed. This BS might be the subjective counterpart of *alogia* as a primary negative symptom and/or *anhedonia* (*asociality*) as a secondary negative symptom, if leading to avoid conversations, that is, to social withdrawal.

Unstable ideas of reference: Subjective, subclinical experience of self-reference for which no explanation outside one's own mental processes is sought, and which is immediately overcome. This BS might be the subjective counterpart of *anhedonia* (*asociality*) as a secondary negative symptom, if leading to social withdrawal.

Disturbances of abstract thinking: Deficits in the comprehension of any kind of abstract, figurative, or symbolic phrases or content as well as a limitation of the ability to go beyond the literal meaning of words, sentences, or phrases.

continued >

Box 2.1 Basic symptom criteria and definitions of relevant symptoms *(Continued)*

COGNITIVE-PERCEPTIVE BASIC SYMPTOMS (COPER)

At least any one of the following ten basic symptoms with a SPI-A or SPI-CY score of at least '3' (i.e. at least weekly occurrence) within the last three months *and* first occurrence at least 12 months ago:

Decreased ability to discriminate between ideas/perception, or fantasy/true memories: A self-recognized difficulty in locating the source of an experience/memory (external vs. internal, mental) that results in an inability to immediately distinguish between current imagination, and real perceptions or memories of real events.

Derealisation: A change in how the person relates emotionally to the environment, which is commonly experienced as an estrangement and detachment from the visual world or, rarely, as an increased emotional affinity for the environment.

Visual perception disturbances (excluding blurred vision, hypersensitivity to light): Misperceptions of visual stimuli while the person is fully aware of their true appearance and, therefore, immediately attributes them to a problem with her/his own eyesight or mental processes.

Acoustic perception disturbances (excluding hypersensitivity to sounds/noises): Misperceptions of acoustic stimuli while the person is fully aware of their true sound and, therefore, immediately attributes the misperceptions to a problem with her/his own hearing or mental processes.

Thought perseveration: A kind of thought interference in which intruding, emotionally neutral, and irrelevant thoughts or images occur repeatedly.

Thought interference (see COGDIS)
Thought pressure (see COGDIS)
Thought blockages (see COGDIS)
Disturbance of receptive speech (see COGDIS)
Unstable ideas of reference (see COGDIS)

Note: A general requirement of BS is their novelty; that is, their report as a disruption in a person's 'normal' self. Self-recognized aberrations in mental processes that have always been present in a trait-like manner can be rated in SPI-A and SPI-CY (rating of '7'), but are not accounted for as BS in the strict sense and, consequently, would not contribute to BS criteria.

More in-depth definitions of BS as well as example questions for the assessment of patients and examples of their statements are provided in the SPI-A and SPI-CY, which can be ordered in various languages from: https://www.fioritieditore.com/en/prodotto/schizophrenia-proneness-instrument-adult-version-spi-a-3/ and https://www.fioritieditore.com/en/prodotto/schizophrenia-proneness-instrument-child-and-youth-spi-cy-extended-english-version-2/.

Adapted from Schultze-Lutter, F., Subjective symptoms of schizophrenia in research and the clinic: the basic symptom concept, *Schizophrenia Bulletin*, 35, 1, pp. 5–8. Copyright (2009) with permission from Oxford University Press. DOI: https://doi.org/10.1093/schbul/sbn139

symptoms—compared to UHR criteria, which were more frequently followed by affective psychoses (Fusar-Poli, Bechdolf, Taylor, et al. 2013).

Recently, a community study of 2683 16- to 40-year-old citizens of the Swiss canton Bern reported that any of the 14 BS included in COPER and or COGDIS was reported by 9.8 per cent of the participants within the three months prior to the telephone interview (Schultze-Lutter, Michel, Ruhrmann, et al. 2018a). Yet, these BS commonly occurred rarely so that the BS criteria's frequency requirement of an occurrence of at least once in a week (see Box 2.1) was only reported by few participants. Consequently, only 2.01 per cent met any one of the two BS psychosis-risk criteria (Schultze-Lutter, et al. 2018a). When the association of BS criteria with the presence of a non-psychotic axis-I disorder and with a functional deficit in terms of a score below 71 on the Social and Occupational Functioning Assessment Scale (APA, 1994) was examined as proxy measures of clinical significance, the presence of BS criteria was significantly related to both. In doing so, the association with a functional deficit (Odds Ratio = 15.9) was considerably stronger than that with a mental disorder (Odds Ratio = 5.4), indicating that BS criteria are not merely an indicator of mental illness but a source of psychosocial functional impairment by themselves (Schultze-Lutter, et al. 2018a). Whether the association between these BS and functional impairment is mediated by negative symptoms and/or BS resembling negative symptoms need to be studied in future.

2.4 Assessments of basic symptoms

Following a first unpublished initial assessment, the Heidelberg Checklist, the *Bonn Scale for the Assessment of Basic Symptoms* (BSABS; Huber, 1986; Gross, Huber, Klosterkötter, et al. 1987) and the *Frankfurt Complaint Questionnaire* (FCQ; Süllwold, 1986; 1991) were developed in parallel—the BSABS as a semi-structured clinical interview on 142 single BS, and the FCQ as a 98-item self-report questionnaire with some BS assessed by multiple items. Both BSABS and FCQ rate only presence/absence but not severity of single BS. Despite the conjoint development of the BSABS and the FCQ, subsequent studies reported poor correspondence between interview-assessed BS and their presumably corresponding counterpart in the FCQ, indicating poor convergent validity of the self-rating of BS in comparison to their gold standard interview assessment (Maß, R., Hitschfeld, K., Wall, et al. 1997; Michel, Kutschal, Schimmelmann, et al. 2017).

Based on multidimensional analyses of BSABS data (Schultze-Lutter, Steinmeyer, Ruhrmann, et al. 2008; Schultze-Lutter, et al. 2012b), the *Schizophrenia Proneness Instruments* were developed in an adult version (SPI-A (Schultze-Lutter, Addington, Ruhrmann, et al. 2007a) and a children and youth version (SPI-CY; Schultze-Lutter, Marshall, and Koch, 2012a; Fux, Walger, Schimmelmann, et al. 2013) as economic BS assessments that also allow rating of severity in terms of frequency.

2.5 Basic symptom dimensions

The SPI-A was generated and validated based on longitudinal and cross-sectional BSABS data using multidimensional scaling analyses (Schultze-Lutter, et al. 2008). The generated six BS dimensions including 34 items exhibited a rather robust structure in adult samples across different states of psychosis, from true pro-dromal to multi-episode states. Their structure even remained largely unchanged when BS assessment turned from a binary assessment of presence to an ordinal assessment of severity. Because this structure could not be replicated in a sample of patients with non-psychotic, depressive disorders, it was concluded that these dimensions were inherent to schizophrenia across different stages of the illness. Thus, they offered a good starting point for the development of the SPI-A, i.e., for the assessment of psychosis-risk symptoms that occur early in course of the illness, thereby serving as valid and reliable subscales (Schultze-Lutter, et al. 2008). Together with a dimension built on criteria-relevant cognitive BS (see Box 2.1), the dimensions 'Affective-Dynamic Disturbances' (incl. impaired toler-ance to certain stressors, a change in general mood, a general decrease in emo-tional responsiveness, and a decrease in positive emotional responsiveness) and 'Cognitive-Attentional Impediments' (including hyperdistractability, inability to divide attention, difficulties with short-term memory, concentration disturbances, slowed-down thinking, and lack of purposive thoughts) formed central dimen-sions of the BS space (see Box 2.2). This indicated that BS phenomenologically resembling observable negative symptoms are a core dimension of psychosis. Perceptive and body perceptive BS as well as some criteria-relevant cognitive BS, however, formed three peripheral dimensions, indicating their role as accessory phenomena (Schultze-Lutter, et al. 2008; Schultze-Lutter, et al. 2012b).

Notwithstanding the stability of the BS dimensions in adult samples, these failed to replicate in a child and adolescent inpatient sample with an onset of psych-osis before the age of 18 (Schultze-Lutter, et al. 2012b). This sample revealed a four-dimensional structure based on 49 items of the BSABS, whereby again a large 'Adynamia' dimension (including BS of the dimensions 'Affective-Dynamic Disturbances' and 'Cognitive-Attentional Impediments' in addition to exhaust-ibility, reduced energy, drive, and persistence as well as affective disturbances, and forgetfulness; see Box 2.2) formed the exclusive core dimension. Thus, this dimension includes several BS that might be regarded as the subjective coun-terpart of observable primary negative symptoms, in particular in terms of avolition or asthenia (see Box 2.2). However, unlike personal vulnerability fac-tors in terms of Janzarik's 'dynamic insufficiency', these BS are decidedly not part of a pre-existing trait-like deficit, that is, of the person's 'normal' self, but only develop in the course of mental disorders (Huber, 1995). Furthermore, unlike Conrad's 'trema' in which similar deficits are observed (also in terms of current primary negative symptoms), these BS are primarily subjective and, thought to occur before the 'trema', might not be observable as long as they do not ex-haust the person's resources to deal with them (Huber, 1995). The other three

Box 2.2 Basic symptoms phenomenologically resembling observable negative symptoms, which were included in the SPI-CY dimension 'Adynamia'

ADYNAMIA

Not part of the BS psychosis-risk criteria, COPER and COGDIS

Reduced energy and vitality: An impairment in strength or power, feeling weak, floppy, or tired, or 'cannot do as many things as I used to'. This BS might be the subjective counterpart of *avolition* as a primary negative symptom.

Reduced persistence, patience: An impairment in perseverance, endurance, or diligence, increased impatience, or a reduced ability to stick with one task or to sit quietly. This BS might be the subjective counterpart of *avolition* as a primary negative symptom.

Reduced drive and initiative: A reduction in motivation, ambition, or determination that is primarily a decrease in drive and initiative, rather than failing to take an interest. This BS might be the subjective counterpart of *avolition* as a primary negative symptom.

Impaired tolerance to certain stressors:[a] A reduced stress tolerance or lack of resilience experienced in response to any kind of labour or to certain situations, or the anticipation of these situations that have not been particularly burdensome before. The prevailing feeling is one of being exhausted or worn out by the respective task or situation, and this is often accompanied by other expressions of impaired stress tolerance, such as: restlessness or nervousness, sleep disturbances, rumination, the inability to mentally 'switch off', concentration disturbances, body perception disturbances, and/or somatic disturbances. The four BS subsumed here might all be the subjective counterpart of *avolition* as a primary negative symptom.

... to physical and/or mental labour: A reduced stress tolerance or lack of resilience in response to daily routine experienced as a general decrease in stress tolerance or resilience that manifests in an increased propensity for physical and mental exhaustion and fatigue, a general lack of strength, weakness, or tiredness, and a feeling of limited ability and efficiency. This BS must be combined with at least one other sign of reduced stress tolerance.

... to unusual, unexpected or specific novel demands:[a] A reduced stress tolerance or lack of resilience experienced in response to extraordinary demands that are not part of the daily routine and are imminent or very recent. This BS is frequently expressed in complaints about not being able to stand out-of-routine situations any more, being stressed-out by them, or feeling the need to avoid them because of anticipating a negative impact on metal state.

... to certain social everyday situations:[a] A reduced stress tolerance or lack of resilience experienced in response to everyday social situations that generally involve a multitude of stimuli but have not previously been regarded as unpleasant or negative. They include: (1) conversations, especially over a longer period or with several persons at once, (2) visiting people, (3) crowds, the hustle and bustle of city or street life, in supermarkets, at public and social events, or on public transport, (4) visual and/or auditory (over-) stimulation, especially by electronic media. This BS might also be the subjective counterpart of *anhedonia* (*asociality*) as a secondary negative symptom if reacting with social withdrawal.

continued >

> **Box 2.2** Basic symptoms phenomenologically resembling observable negative symptoms, which were included in the SPI-CY dimension 'Adynamia' *(Continued)*
>
> **... to working under pressure of time or rapidly changing different demands:**[a] This BS is a reduced ability to carry out a task within a reasonable time, or to deal with rapidly changing tasks. Affected persons report that they have difficulties coping with time pressure (hectic, rushing), and experience time-sensitive tasks as unbearable, exhausting, or confusing.
>
> **Change in mood:**[a] A change in underlying mood that occurs spontaneously, is unrelated to negative events, is perceived as uncontrollable, and is different from temporary fluctuations of affect known from 'healthy' times.
>
> **Change in emotional responsiveness:**[a] A reduced or missing ability to experience both positive and negative emotions, or, in extreme cases, a 'feeling of loss of feelings'. This BS might be the subjective counterpart of *affective flattening* as a primary negative symptom.
>
> **Decrease in positive emotional responsiveness towards others:**[a] A reduced ability to experience positive emotions, while the experience of negative emotions is not impaired. This BS might be the subjective counterpart of *affective flattening* as a primary negative symptom.
>
> **Intermittent, recurrent depressive mood swings:** Periods of low or depressive mood that occur without a recognizable reason (though at rare times a triggering event might be discernible) and remit spontaneously.
>
> **Disturbance in presenting oneself:** A disturbance of the availability of and control over the repertoire of non-verbal expression, especially gestures, facial expressions, glances, and voice modulation. The persons feel that they have—at least temporarily—lost the ability to express themselves non-verbally. This BS might be the subjective counterpart of *affective flattening* as a primary negative symptom.
>
> **Increased emotional reactivity in response to everyday events:** Everyday events that had not been previously associated with any strong or persisting emotional reaction are now upsetting. Usually they are experienced as causing agitation, inner restlessness, and tension, and lead to depressive ruminations or an inability to turn one's mind off the event.
>
> **Increased emotional reactivity in response to routine social interactions that affect the young person directly or indirectly:** A self-experienced hypersensitivity to daily events, involving the person, or his or her relatives or friends. In comparison to the premorbid phase, the person feels as if he or she has become 'thin-skinned' and is more easily moved or offended. It is essential that the person knows that he or she is over-reacting.
>
> **Difficulties concentrating:**[b] Difficulties with concentration, in terms of having problems maintaining attention over time without being distracted or drifting off. This BS might be the subjective counterpart of *attentional impairment* as a primary negative symptom.
>
> **Forgetfulness, scatterbrainedness:** Memory disturbances that cannot be assigned to working, short-, or long-term memory but rather affect implicit learning and retrieval of related memory contents. This BS might manifest itself in frequently losing or looking for things. This BS might be the subjective counterpart of *attentional impairment* as a primary negative symptom.

Box 2.2 Basic symptoms phenomenologically resembling observable
negative symptoms, which were included in the SPI-CY dimension 'Adynamia'
(Continued)

Slowed-down thinking:[b] The experience of slowness in thinking in terms of a
general sense that thinking has become slower and harder, irrespective of the difficulty
level of the task. This BS might be the subjective counterpart of avolition as a primary
negative symptom. This BS might be the subjective counterpart of *avolition* and/or
alogia as primary negative symptoms.

Lack of 'thought energy' or goal-directed thoughts:[b] A disturbance of
initiating thought, or a lack 'thought energy' or intellectual purpose, experienced an
impaired ability to initiate, plan, and structure certain actions such as cooking or active
participating in a conversation. This BS might be the subjective counterpart of *avolition*
as a primary negative symptom and *anhedonia (asociality)* as a secondary negative
symptom if reacting with social withdrawal.

[a] included in the SPI-A dimension 'Affective-Dynamic Disturbances'

[b] included in the SPI-A dimension 'Cognitive-Attentional Impediments'

Note: A general requirement of BS is their novelty, that is, their report as a disruption in a person's
'normal' self. Self-recognized aberrations in mental processes that have always been present in a
trait-like manner can be rated in SPI-A and SPI-CY (rating of '7'), but are not accounted for as BS in
the strict sense.

More in-depth definitions of BS as well as example questions for the assessment of patients and
examples of their statements are provided in the SPI-A and SPI-CY, which can be ordered in various
languages from: https://www.fioritieditore.com/en/prodotto/schizophrenia-proneness-instrument-
adult-version-spi-a-3/ and https://www.fioritieditore.com/en/prodotto/schizophrenia-proneness-
instrument-child-and-youth-spi-cy-extended-english-version-2/.

Source data from: Schimmelmann, B. G. and Schultze-Lutter, F., *European Child and Adolescent
Psychiatry*, 21(5), Early detection and intervention of psychosis in children and adolescents:
urgent need for studies, pp. 239–41. © Springer-Verlag 2012. Doi: https://doi.org/10.1007/
s00787-012-0271-z

---

dimensions 'Neuroticism', 'Perception Disturbances', and 'Thought and Motor
Disturbances'—the latter two including the 14 criteria-relevant cognitive and perceptive BS—formed the peripheral dimensions (Schultze-Lutter, et al. 2012b).

The important role of 'Adynamia' in children and adolescents was further
supported in the SPI-CY pilot study (Fux, Walger, Schimmelmann, et al. 2013).
Therein, psychosis-risk patients according to UHR and/or BS criteria scored
higher than clinical and healthy controls, with the latter scoring lowest in all SPI-
CY dimensions. Pairwise subscale differences indicated at least moderate group
effects (Rosenthal's $r \geq 0.37$), which were largest for 'Adynamia' ($0.52 \leq r \geq$
0.70). This outstanding role of 'Adynamia' was broadly in line with studies using
the BSABS in adolescent early-onset psychosis and clinical control patients, and
community controls (Resch, Parzer, and Amminger, 1998; Meng, Schimmelmann,
Koch, et al. 2009). These found the BSABS category 'Direct Minus Symptoms', a

main source of 'Adynamia' items, to be second-best in discriminating the psychosis patients from the other groups. The BSABS category discriminating best between groups was 'Cognitive Disturbances' that also includes the non-specific cognitive BS that are part of 'Adynamia in the SPI-CY (see Box 2.2). Thus, six of the top ten BS discriminating between groups are part of 'Adynamia (impaired tolerance to physical/mental labour and certain social everyday situations, change in basic mood and emotional responsiveness, difficulties concentrating, and slowed thinking). The other four discriminative BS (thought interference and perseveration, decreased ability to discriminate between ideas/perception, or fantasy/true memories, and decreased capacity to discriminate between different kinds of emotions) are part of the 'Thought and Motor Disturbances' of the SPI-CY (Meng, et al. 2009).

In contrast, however, a comparison of SPI-A-assessed BS in adult samples of psychosis-risk patients, patients with first-episode schizophrenia, and patients with a depressive disorder (Schultze-Lutter, Ruhrmann, Picker, et al. 2007c) found the SPI-A dimension 'Affective-Dynamic Disturbances' (see Box 2.2) least discriminative between the depressive and the other groups. A similar result had earlier been reported from a study that compared adult ICD-10 (International Statistical Classification of Diseases and Health Problems, 10th revision) diagnostic categories and healthy controls using the BSABS (Klosterkötter, et al. 1996). In this study, too, schizophrenic disorders (F2) were least distinguished from other groups by subjective deficits in drive, initiative, stress tolerance, emotional responsiveness and control, concentration, and thought energy and initiative (Klosterkötter, et al. 1996).

Taken together, these studies indicate that BS as included in the SPI-CY dimension of 'Adynamia' might be even more characteristic for early-onset psychosis for that a greater burden of negative symptoms in comparison to adult-onset psychosis has been described (Puig, Baeza, de la Serna, et al. 2017).

2.6 Basic symptoms and schizotypy

By definition, BS differ from what patients consider to be their *normal* mental self and functions; moreover, being state phenomena, they commonly fluctuate, mostly in response to stress. This makes BS distinct from trait-like schizotypy features considered as part of the *normal* self and being commonly stable over time. Furthermore, as both healthy offspring of schizophrenics (Tarbox and Pogue-Geile, 2011; Tarbox, Almasy, Gur, et al. 2012) and psychosis-risk individuals according to UHR or BS criteria (Flückiger, Ruhrmann, Debbané, et al. 2016) were marked by below-average positive-trait schizotypy, and as BS criteria were not predicted by schizotypy expression (Flückiger, et al. 2016), BS cannot merely be regarded as exacerbated states of a mental condition that has always been there at the trait level. This state-trait distinction of schizotypy dimensions and BS was recently supported by a 1-year follow-up study that showed significant changes in the 14 criteria-relevant BS and UHR symptoms, but not in positive and negative schizotypy with no significant correlation of difference scores between schizotypy and BS scores (Michel, Flückiger, Kindler, et al. 2019).

Similar to the BS concept, the schizotypy concept also considers a benign course, especially in the absence of negative schizotypy and cognitive symptoms (Mason, 2014; Barrantes-Vidal, Grant, and Kwapil, 2015; Debbané, Eliez, Badoud, et al. 2015; Grant, Green, and Mason, 2018). This view was recently confirmed by structural equation modelling in a sample from two early detection services (Flückiger, Michel, Grant, et al. 2019). The model revealed that much of the relation between negative schizotypy (physical and social anhedonia as assessed by the Wisconsin Schizotypy Scales; Chapman, Chapman, and Raulin, 1976; Eckblad, Chapman, Chapman, et al. 1982) and negative symptoms as assessed with the Structured Interview for Psychosis-Risk Syndromes (SIPS; McGlashan, Walsh, and Woods, 2010) was mainly mediated by the additional symptom load of criteria-relevant cognitive BS described in Box 2.1. The relation between positive schizotypy (magical ideation and perceptual aberrations; Chapman, Chapman, and Raulin, 1978; Eckblad and Chapman, 1983) and attenuated positive symptoms was also mediated by cognitive BS, though the direct path between both measures was stronger than the mediated path (Flückiger, et al. 2019).

The strong mediator role of cognitive BS in the relation of negative schizotypy and negative symptoms is significant as current models of schizotypy (Claridge, 1997) regard positive schizotypy and disease-proneness as constituting different dimensions (Grant, Green, and Mason, 2018), whereby the cognitive-disorganized and negative dimensions constitute disease-proneness. In fact, proponents of these models (Grant, 2015a; 2015b; Mohr and Claridge, 2015) argue that the difference between so-called happy schizotypes and patients with schizophrenia spectrum disorders is not one of quantity or severity of psychosis proneness but one of quality of phenomena. These qualitative differences are due to influences of other dimensions that are more closely linked to negative and disorganized schizotypy (Barrantes-Vidal, Grant, and Kwapil, 2015; Grant, 2015a; 2015b; Mohr and Claridge, 2015; Grant, et al. 2018). Being distinct from continuously distributed schizotypy, schizophrenia is thus, regarded as a breakdown process and endpoint on a second graded continuum that starts from schizotypal personality disorder (Grant, et al. 2018). Thus, positive schizotypy in itself might as well be beneficial, as it was associated with personal well-being, flexible and unconventional thinking, favourable personality traits, and psychological features such as openness to experience, fantasy proneness, and spirituality (Mohr and Claridge, 2015). In contrast to the continuum hypothesis of psychosis focusing on positive schizotypy, high negative schizotypy that was found to be predictive of attenuated psychotic symptoms and, in psychosis-risk samples, of conversion to psychosis (Flückiger, et al. 2016) and/or high disorganized schizotypy seem to be most relevant to poor functioning and mental ill-health (Mohr and Claridge, 2015). Recently, the view on the negative dimension was further sharpened by a study (Fumero, Marrero, and Fonseca-Pedrero, 2018) showing different negative effects of negative and disorganized features of schizotypal personality disorder on happiness, life satisfaction, affect, and all aspects of well-being. Of the positive dimension, only ideas of reference and suspiciousness were significantly associated with poor autonomy, and negative affect and poor environmental mastery, respectively. Other positive features were either associated with positive effects or unrelated to these outcomes (Fumero, et al. 2018). Taken together, these findings point towards negative schizotypy and cognitive BS as early treatment targets when trying to prevent (attenuated) negative symptoms from developing or progressing. The potential mediating role of BS phenomenologically more similar to negative symptoms (that is BS included in the SPI-A subscales 'Attentional-Dynamic Disturbances' and 'Cognitive-Attentional Impediments', and the SPI-CY subscale 'Adynamia', respectively) between negative schizotypy and negative symptoms has not been studied so far.

2.7 Basic symptoms, (attenuated) positive and negative symptoms

For their spontaneous, immediate recognition by patients as disturbances of their own (mental) processes, BS are distinct from the (attenuated) positive symptoms that define the UHR criteria and frank psychosis, in which reality testing is disturbed, at least to some degree. In addition, BS are also mostly phenomenologically distinct from these symptoms because they are not necessarily observable by others in terms of odd thinking, disturbed speech, and formal thought disorder, and are not defined by culturally abnormal ideas, such as unusual thought contents (e.g. magical thinking, ideas of reference, paranoid ideation, suspiciousness, and other delusions), and 'Ich-Störungen' (i.e. thought broadcasting, insertion, withdrawal, and delusion of alien control). Neither are BS related to the outside world, thus being distinct from hallucinations.

A recent network analysis of the altogether 86 symptoms assessed with the SPI-A, the SIPS and the Positive and Negative Symptoms Scale (PANSS; Kay, Fiszbein, and Opler, 1987) confirmed the slightly different nature of self-experienced BS and more observable positive, negative, and other associated symptoms on the one hand and their close relation on the other (Jimeno, Gomez-Pilar, Poza, et al., in press). It revealed a single dense network of highly interrelated symptoms with five discernible symptom subgroups. In line with current diagnostic emphasis on positive symptoms, disorganized communication was the most central symptom, followed by delusions and hallucinations. In line with the BS model, the network was distinguished by symptom severity running from SPI-A via SIPS to PANSS assessments. The main amalgamation of scales was between the corresponding and strongly connected positive symptoms of SIPS and PANSS. Despite the network's density, based on the position and nature of symptoms, five partly overlapping symptom subgroups were discernible with positive, negative, and cognitive-disorganized symptoms forming the core, and (body) perception and affective symptoms building the periphery. Next to negative and some general symptoms of SIPS and PANSS, the negative subgroup also included the three non-affective BS of 'Affective-Dynamic Disturbances', reinforcing their phenom- enological closeness to these. These lay in close proximity to the two affective BS of this dimension that were part of the affective subgroup, and to two of the unspecific cognitive BS of 'Attentional-Cognitive Impairments'. As regards symp- toms that were influencing or 'bridging' the different subgroups and, thus, can be considered as most relevant treatment targets, difficulty in abstract thinking (PANSS-N5) of the cognitive-disorganized subgroup and, of the negative sub- group, stereotyped thinking (PANSS-N7) and poor rapport (PANSS-N3) were significantly correlated to a variety of positive features, indicating their signifi- cant role in maintaining positive symptoms. Additionally, however, the negative symptoms blunted affect (PANSS-N1), emotional withdrawal (PANSS-N2), so- cial anhedonia (SIPS-N1), and deterioration in role functioning (SIPS-N6) showed similar links to the positive dimension. The affective peripheral PANSS items de- pression (G6) was mainly, though still weakly, linked to the negative dimension by avolition (SIPS-N2) and passive social withdrawal (PANSS-N4). The affective subgroup was linked to the positive subgroup mainly by excitement (PANSS-P4), indicating that high excitement (PANSS-P4)—if not treated early—might trigger exacerbation of positive symptoms.

2.8 Conclusion

On the one hand, BS, in particular those included in the SPI-CY subscale 'Adynamia' and related subscales of the SPI-A, can be regarded as very mild, subthreshold, not yet observable forms of negative symptoms and thus a source of primary negative symptoms. On the other hand, other BS, including those used for the prediction of psychosis, might evoke secondary negative symptoms (Kirschner, Aleman, and Kaiser, 2017) as a result of inadequate coping with these BS. In any case, gaining a better understanding of the origins of negative symp- toms by assessing BS will help better titrating pharmacological and psychological treatment.

REFERENCES

American Psychiatric Association (1994). *Diagnostic and Statistical Manual of Mental Disorders*, 4th edn. Washington, DC, American Psychiatric Association.

Barrantes-Vidal, N., Grant, P., Kwapil, T. R. (2015). The role of schizotypy in the study of the etiology of schizophrenia spectrum disorders. *Schizophrenia Bulletin*, **41**(suppl 2), S408–S416. doi: 10.1093/schbul/sbu191.

Chapman, L. J., Chapman, J. P., Raulin, M. L. (1976). Scales for physical and social anhedonia. *Journal of Abnormal Psychology*, **85**, 374–82.

Chapman, L. J., Chapman, J. P., Raulin, M. L. (1978). Body-image aberration in schizophrenia. *Journal of Abnormal Psychology*, **87**(4), 399–407.

Claridge, G. (1997). 'Theoretical background' in G Claridge (ed.), *Schizotypy: Implications for Illness and Health*. Oxford, Oxford University Press, pp. 1–7.

Debbané, M., Eliez, S., Badoud, D., Conus, P., Flückiger, R., Schultze-Lutter, F. (2015). Developing psychosis and its risk states through the lens of schizotypy. *Schizophrenia Bulletin*, **41**(suppl 2), S396–S407. doi: 10.1093/schbul/sbu176.

Eckblad, M., Chapman, L. J., Chapman, J. P., Mishlove, M. (1982). *The Revised Social Anhedonia Scale*. Madison, University of Wisconsin.

Eckblad, M., Chapman, L. J. (1983). Magical ideation as an indicator of schizotypy. *Journal of Consulting and Clinical Psychology*, **51**(2), 215–25.

Fumero, A., Marrero, R. J., Fonseca-Pedrero, E. (2018). Well-being in schizotypy: The effect of subclinical psychotic experiences. *Psicothema*, **30**(2), 177–82. doi: 10.7334/psicothema2017.100.

Eisner, E., Drake, R., Lobban, F., Bucci, S., Emsley, R., Barrowclough, C. (2018). Comparing early signs and basic symptoms as methods for predicting psychotic relapse in clinical practice. *Schizophrenia Research*, 192, 124–30. doi: 10.1016/j.schres.2017.04.050.

Flückiger, R., Ruhrmann, S., Debbané, M., Michel, C., Hubl, D., Schimmelmann, B. G., et al. (2016). Psychosis-predictive value of self-reported schizotypy in a clinical high risk sample. *Journal of Abnormal Psychology*, **125**(7), 923–8. doi: 10.1037/abn0000192.

Flückiger, R., Michel, C., Grant, P., Ruhrmann, S., Vogeley, K., Hubl, D., et al. (2019). The interrelationship between schizotypy, clinical high risk for psychosis and related symptoms: cognitive disturbances matter. *Schizophrenia Research*, 210, 188–9. doi: 10.1016/j.schres.2018.12.039.

Fusar-Poli, P., Bechdolf, A., Taylor, M. J., Bonoldi, I., Carpenter, W. T., Yung, A. R., et al. (2013). At risk for schizophrenic or affective psychoses? A meta-analysis of DSM/ICD diagnostic outcomes in individuals at high clinical risk. *Schizophrenia Bulletin*, **39**(4), 923–32. doi: 10.1093/schbul/sbs060.

Fux, L., Walger, P., Schimmelmann, B. G., Schultze-Lutter, F. (2013). The Schizophrenia Proneness Instrument, Child and Youth version (SPI-CY): practicability and discriminative validity. *Schizophrenia Research*, **146**(1–3), 69–78. doi: 10.1016/j.schres.2013.02.014.

Gaebel, W., Riesbeck, M. (2014). Are there clinically useful predictors and early warning signs for pending relapse? *Schizophrenia Research*, **152**, 469–77. doi: 10.1016/j.schres.2013.08.003.

Grant, P. (2015a). Is schizotypy per se a suitable endophenotype of schizophrenia?—do not forget to distinguish positive from negative facets. *Frontiers in Psychiatry*, 6. doi:10.3389/fpsyt.2015.00143.

Grant, P. (2015b). 'Genetic associations: the basis of schizotypy' in G. Claridge, O. Mason (eds), *Schizotypy: New Dimensions*. London, Routledge; pp. 48–61.

Grant, P., Green, M. J., Mason, O. (2018). Models of schizotypy. The importance of conceptual clarity. *Schizophrenia Bulletin*, **44**(suppl 2), S556–63. doi: 10.1093/schbul/sby012.

Gross, G., Huber, G. (1989). Das Basissymptomkonzept idiopathischer Psychosen. *Zentralblatt für Neurologie und Psychiatrie*, **252**, 655–73.

Gross, G., Huber, G., Klosterkötter, J., Linz, M. (1987). *Bonner Skala für die Beurteilung von Basissymptomen (BSABS; Bonn Scale for the Assessment of Basic Symptoms)*. Berlin, Springer-Verlag.

CHAPTER 2

Huber, G. (1986). 'Psychiatrische Aspekte des Basisstörungskonzepts' in L. Süllwold, G. Huber (Hrsg.). *Schizophrene Basisstörungen*. Berlin, Springer, pp. 39–143.

Huber, G. (1966). Reine Defektsyndrome und Basisstadien endogener Psychose. *Fortschritte der Neurologie-Psychiatrie*, **34**, 409–26.

Huber, G. (1995). Prodrome der Schizophrenie. *Fortschritte der Neurologie-Psychiatrie*, **63**(4), 131–8. doi: 10.1055/s-2007-996611.

Jimeno, N., Gomez-Pilar, J., Poza, J., Hornero, R., Vogeley, K., Meisenzahl, E., et al. Main symptomatic treatment targets in suspected and early psychosis: new insights from network analysis. *Schizophrenia Bulletin*, in press.

Kay, S. R., Fiszbein, A., Opler, L. A. (1987). The Positive and Negative Syndrome Scale (PANSS) for schizophrenia. *Schizophrenia Bulletin*, **13**, 261–76.

Kirschner, M., Aleman, A., Kaiser, S. (2017). Secondary negative symptoms—a review of mechanisms, assessment and treatment. *Schizophrenia Research*, **186**, 29–38. doi: 10.1016/j.schres.2016.05.003.

Klosterkötter, J., Ebel, H., Schultze-Lutter, F., Steinmeyer, E. M. (1996). Diagnostic validity of basic symptoms. *European Archives of Psychiatry and Clinical Neuroscience*, **246**, 147–54.

Klosterkötter, J., Hellmich, M., Steinmeyer, E. M., Schultze-Lutter, F. (2001). Diagnosing schizophrenia in the initial prodromal phase. *Archives in General Psychiatry*, **58**, 158–64.

Klosterkötter, J., Gross, G., Huber, G., Wieneke, A., Steinmeyer, E. M., Schultze-Lutter, F. (1997). Evaluation of the 'Bonn Scale for the Assessment of Basic Symptoms—BSABS' as an instrument for the assessment of schizophrenia proneness: A review of recent findings. *Neurology, Psychiatry and Brain Research*, **5**, 137–50.

Marder, S. R., Galderisi, S. (2017). The current conceptualization of negative symptoms in schizophrenia. *World Psychiatry*, **16**, 14–24. doi: 10.1002/wps.20385.

Mason, O. J. (2014). The duality of schizotypy: is it both dimensional and categorical? *Frontiers in Psychiatry*, **5**, 134. doi:10.3389/fpsyt.2014.00134.

Maß, R., Hitschfeld, K., Wall, E., Wagner, H. B. (1997). Validität der Erfassung schizophrener Basissymptome. *Der Nervenarzt*, **68**(30), 205–11.

Mayer-Gross, W. (1932). 'Die Schizophrenie. Die Klinik' in O. Bumke (ed.). *Handbuch der Geisteskrankheiten—Spezieller Teil V: Die Schizophrenie*. Berlin, Springer, pp. 293–578.

McGlashan, T. H., Walsh, B., Woods, S. (2010). *The Psychosis-Risk Syndrome. Handbook for Diagnosis and Follow-Up*. New York, Oxford University Press.

Mohr, C., Claridge, G. (2015). Schizotypy—do not worry, it is not all worrisome. *Schizophrenia Bulletin*, **41**(suppl 2), S436–S443. doi: 10.1093/schbul/sbu185.

Meng, H., Schimmelmann, B. G., Koch, E., Bailey, B., Parzer, P., Günter, M., et al. (2009). Basic symptoms in the general population and in psychotic and nonpsychotic psychiatric adolescents. *Schizophrenia Research*, **111**(1–3), 32–8. doi: 10.1016/j.schres.2009.03.001.

Michel, C., Kutschal, C., Schimmelmann, B. G., Schultze-Lutter, F. (2017). Convergent and concurrent validity of the Frankfurt Complaint Questionnaire as a screener for psychosis risk. *Journal of Risk Research*, **20**(11), 1480–96. doi: 10.1080/13669877.2016.1179209.

Michel, C., Flückiger, R., Kindler, J., Hubl, D., Kaess, M., Schultze-Lutter, F. (2019). The trait-state distinction of schizotypy and clinical high risk: results from a 1-year follow-up. *World Psychiatry*, **18**(1), 108–9. doi: 10.1002/wps.20595.

Parnas, J., Møller, P., Kircher, T., Thalbitzer, J., Jansson, L., Handest, P., et al. (2005). EASE: Examination of Anomalous Self-Experience. *Psychopathology*, **38**(5), 236–58. doi 10.1159/000088441.

Puig, O., Baeza, I., de la Serna, E., Cabrera, B., Mezquida, G., Bioque, M., et al. (2017). Persistent negative symptoms in first-episode psychosis: early cognitive and social functioning correlates and differences between early and adult onset. *Journal of Clinical Psychiatry*, **78**(9), 1414–22. doi: 10.4088/JCP.16m11122.

Resch, F., Parzer, P., Amminger, G. P. (1998). On the existence of early warning signs of schizophrenic syndromes among children and adolescents. *Neurology, Psychiatry and Brain Research*, **6**, 45–50.

Schimmelmann, B. G., Michel, C., Martz-Irngartinger, A., Linder, C., Schultze-Lutter, F. (2015). Age matters in the prevalence and clinical significance of ultra-high-risk for psychosis symptoms and criteria in the general population: findings from the BEAR and BEARS-Kid studies. *World Psychiatry*, **14**, 189–97. doi: 10.1002/wps.20216.

Schmidt, S. J., Schultze-Lutter, F., Bendall, S., Groth, N., Inderbitzin, N., Michel, C., et al. (2017). Mediators linking childhood adversities and trauma to suicidality in individuals at risk for psychosis. *Frontiers in Psychiatry*, **8**, 242. doi: 10.3389/fpsyt.2017.00242.

Schultze-Lutter, F. (2009). Subjective symptoms of schizophrenia in research and the clinic: the basic symptom concept. *Schizophrenia Bulletin*, **35**, 5–8. doi:10.1093/schbul/sbn139.

Schultze-Lutter, F., Theodoridou, A. (2017). The concept of basic symptoms: its relevance in research and the clinic. *World Psychiatry*, **16**(1), 104–5. doi: 10.1002/wps.20404.

Schultze-Lutter, F., Ruhrmann, S., Klosterkötter, J. (2006). 'Can schizophrenia be predicted phenomenologically?' in J. O. Johannessen, B. Martindale, J. Cullberg (eds). *Evolving Psychosis. Different Stages, Different Treatments*. London, Routledge, pp. 104–23.

Schultze-Lutter, F., Marshall, M., Koch, E. (2012a). *Schizophrenia Proneness Instrument, Child and Youth version; extended English translation (SPI-CY EET)*. Rome: Giovanni Fioriti Editore s.r.l.

Schultze-Lutter, F., Addington, J., Ruhrmann, S., Klosterkötter, J. (2007a). *Schizophrenia Proneness Instrument, Adult version (SPI-A)*. Rome, Giovanni Fioriti Editore s.r.l.

Schultze-Lutter, F., Steinmeyer, E., Ruhrmann, S., Klosterkötter, J. (2008). The dimensional structure of self-reported prodromal disturbances in schizophrenia. *Clinical Neuropsychiatry*, **5**(3), 140–50. https://www.clinicalneuropsychiatry.org/download/no-3-june-2008-the-dimensional-structure-of-self-reported-prodromal-disturbances-in-schizophrenia/

Schultze-Lutter, F., Michel, C., Ruhrmann, S., Schimmelmann, B. G. (2018a). Prevalence and clinical relevance of interview-assessed psychosis risk symptoms in the young adult community. *Psychological Medicine*, **48**, 1167–78. doi: 10.1017/S0033291717002586.

Schultze-Lutter, F., Klosterkötter, J., Picker, H., Steinmeyer, E. M., Ruhrmann, S. (2007b). Predicting first-episode psychosis by basic symptom criteria. *Clinical Neuropsychiatry*, **4**(1), 11–22. https://www.clinicalneuropsychiatry.org/download/no-1-february-2007-predicting-first-episode-psychosis-by-basic-symptom-criteria/.

Schultze-Lutter, F., Ruhrmann, S., Picker, H., Graf von Reventlow, H., Brockhaus-Dumke, A., Klosterkötter, J. (2007c). Basic symptoms in early psychotic and depressive disorders. *British Journal of Psychiatry*, **191**(suppl 51), s31–s37. doi: 10.1192/bjp.191.51.s31.

CHAPTER 2

Schultze-Lutter, F., Ruhrmann, S., Fusar-Poli, P., Bechdolf, A., Schimmelmann, B. G., Klosterkötter, J. (2012b). Basic symptoms and the prediction of first-episode psychosis. *Current Pharmaceutical Design*, **18**(4), 351–7.

Schultze-Lutter, F., Michel, C., Schmidt, S. J., Schimmelmann, B. G., Maric, N. P., Salokangas, R. K. R., et al. (2015). EPA guidance on the early detection of clinical high risk states of psychosis. *European Psychiatry*, **30**, 405–16. doi: 10.1016/j.eurpsy.2015.01.010.

Schultze-Lutter, F., Debbané, M., Theodoridou, A., Wood, S. J., Raballo, A., Michel, C., et al. (2016). Revisiting the basic symptom concept: towards translating risk symptoms for psychosis into neurobiological targets. *Frontiers in Psychiatry*, **7**(9). doi: 10.3389/fpsyt.2016.00009.

Schultze-Lutter, F., Ruhrmann, S., Michel, C., Kindler, J., Schimmelmann, B. G., Schmidt, S. J. (2018b). Age effects on basic symptoms in the community: a route to gain new insight into the neurodevelopment of psychosis? *European Archives of Psychiatry and Clinical Neuroscience*, doi: 10.1007/s00406-018-0949-4.

Süllwold, L. (1986). 'Die Selbstwahrnehmung defizitärer Störungen. Psychologische Aspekte des Basisstörungskonzepts' in L. Süllwold, G. Huber (Hrsg.). *Schizophrene Basisstörungen*. Berlin, Springer, pp. 1–38.

Süllwold, L. (1991). *Manual zum Frankfurter Beschwerde-Fragebogen (FBF)*. Berlin, Springer.

Tarbox, S. I., Pogue-Geile, M. F. (2011). A multivariate perspective on schizotypy and familial association with schizophrenia: a review. *Clinical Psychology Review*, **31**(7), 1169–82. doi: 10.1016/j.cpr.2011.07.002.

Tarbox, S. I., Almasy, L., Gur, R. E., Nimgaonkar, V. L., Pogue-Geile, M. F. (2012). The nature of schizotypy among multigenerational multiplex schizophrenia families. *Journal of Abnormal Psychology*, **121**(2), 396–406. doi: 10.1037/a0026787.

Yung, A. R., Phillips, L. J., McGorry, P. D., McFarlane, C. A., Francey, S., Harrigan, S., et al. (1998). Prediction of psychosis: A step towards indicated prevention of schizophrenia. *British Journal of Psychiatry*, **172**(s33), 14–20. doi: 10.1192/S0007125000297602.

CHAPTER 3

Long-term course of negative symptoms in schizophrenia

Anatoly Smulevich and Dmitry Romanov

KEY POINTS

- Negative symptoms in schizophrenia should be evaluated in a close relation to positive symptoms both in a long-term disease course (prospectively/retrospectively) and at a single point in time (cross-sectionally).
- Regarding the long-term disease course, two types of interaction between negative and positive symptoms could be distinguished: (1) relatively synchronized; and (2) relatively desynchronized trajectory type.
- Synchronization of negative and positive symptoms is characterized by their unidirectional long-term course with the coincident increase of severity in the active period of schizophrenia.
- Desynchronization of negative and positive symptoms is characterized by their bidirectional long-term relations: (1) negative schizophrenia with minimal positive symptoms at the beginning of the disease and further progression of negative symptoms; or (2) schizophrenia with negative symptoms 'that stopped at the very beginning': increasing negative symptoms at the initial stage and no or minimal further increase, while the later course of the disease is characterized by positive symptoms.
- Considering every single time point of the long-term relationship between negative and positive symptoms (cross-sectionally), we describe the concept of 'mutual/common syndromes' at different stages of schizophrenia: initial stage and late stage (residual deficit states).

3.1 Introduction

The beginning of studies on negative symptoms and their association with positive symptoms dates back to the nineteenth century. The credit for introducing the term 'negative symptoms' belongs to H. J. Jackson (1889). According to Jackson, negative symptoms resulted from the impairment of phylogenetically 'younger' brain structures and deficiency of their function that consistently led to manifestation of positive symptoms due to functional release of disinhibited 'older' structures. E. Kraepelin (1915) regarded the deficit symptoms, such as cognitive deterioration, blunted affect, avolition, and loss of energy, as the main clinical phenomena to establish the diagnosis of dementia praecox, not positive symptoms.

The contemporary approach to negative symptoms and their associations with positive symptoms has been strongly influenced by the model of schizophrenia suggested by E. Bleuler (1911). Bleuler considered negative symptoms, such as abnormality of speech, affective incongruence, and autism, as a consequence of the fundamental biological process, and called them 'fundamental symptoms' which, in fact, reflected the manifestations of deficits associated with schizophrenia. Whereas positive phenomena, such as delusions and hallucinations, were defined by Bleuler as 'accessory symptoms'.

Further development of the concept of primary (negative) phenomena, determined by the fundamental biological process, took place in the context of the basic schizophrenic deficit concepts suggested subsequently, for example 'primary insufficiency' (Berze, 1914; Conrad, 1958), 'basic symptoms', and 'pure deficit' (Huber, 1966; 1995), and modern dimensional construct of primary or persistent negative symptoms (Galderisi, et al. 2013; Mucci, Merlotti, Üçok, et al. 2017).[1]

It should also be noted that along with persistent or primary negative symptoms in schizophrenia, there is a set of so-called secondary negative symptoms due to depression, medication side effects, social deprivation, or substance abuse. However, because secondary negative symptoms are common, they can have a major impact on patient-relevant outcomes and can contribute to an integrated model of negative symptoms (Kirschner, Aleman, Kaiser, 2017) (Fig. 3.1). However, a discussion of the course of secondary negative symptoms is not an objective of this chapter (see Chapter 1).

This chapter presents the state-of-the-art concepts—including our contribution (Smulevich, 2016; Smulevich, Romanov, Mukhorina, et al. 2017a; Smulevich, Romanov, Voronova, et al. 2017b; Smulevich, Dubnitskaya, Lobanova, et al. 2018; Smulevich, Kharkova, Lobanova, et al. 2019)—on the relationship of primary negative symptoms with positive symptoms.

The two most important aspects of the discussed topic are:

(1) interrelations of negative and positive symptoms in the long-term course of the disease;

(2) the clinical structure of 'mutual' or 'common syndromes', concomitantly consisting of negative and positive symptoms, described cross-sectionally at different stages of the course of schizophrenia, including the initial period and residual deficit states.

3.2 Long-term course of negative and positive symptoms in schizophrenia

The possibility of multidirectional dynamic of negative compared to positive dimensions was described in various concepts of negative schizophrenia

---

[1] 'Persistent negative symptoms', i.e. affective flattening, alogia, avolition, asociality, correspond to Bleuler's phenomenology of fundamental symptoms.

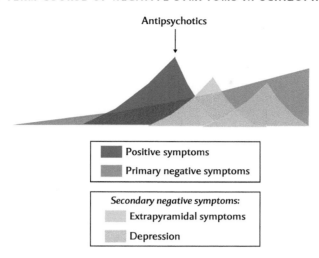

Figure 3.1 Time relations between primary negative, positive, and secondary negative symptoms.

(Crow, 1980; Andreasen and Olsen, 1982; Trimble, 1986; Carpenter, Heinrichs, and Wagman, 1988; Sass, 1989; Mosolov, Potapov, Ushakov, et al. 2014). Furthermore, negative (or deficit) schizophrenia has been defined as a distinct form of the disease, different from 'positive' schizophrenia in neurophysiological parameters and structural anomalies discovered in neuroimaging studies (Delamillieure, Fernandez, Constans, et al. 2000; Nkam, Thibaut, Denise, et al. 2001; Delamillieure, Constans, Fernandez, et al. 2004; Voineskos, Foussias, Lerch, et al. 2013).

Recent research from the Scientific Centre for Mental Health and the Department of Psychiatry and Psychosomatics of the First Moscow State Medical University (Sechenov Medical University) provided evidence that the trajectory of negative schizophrenia, comprising polar tendencies in the development of negative and positive dimensions, represented only one particular case of the interrelations of negative and positive symptoms (e.g. Smulevich, 2016; Smulevich, Romanov, Mukhorina, et al. 2017a; Smulevich, Romanov, Voronova, et al. 2017b; Smulevich, Dubnitskaya, Lobanova, et al. 2018). Two types of long-term course of negative and positive dimensions can be distinguished based on their generally simultaneous or independent progression: (1) a relatively synchronized or simultaneously-progressive trajectory type; and (2) a relatively desynchronized or independently progressive trajectory type, respectively.

3.2.1 Relatively synchronized trajectory of negative and positive symptoms

The relatively synchronized (or simultaneously progressive) trajectory of negative and positive symptoms is characterized by their unidirectional progressive long-term course with the simultaneous increase of severity at the active stage of schizophrenia (see Fig. 3.2). This accords with Snezhnevsky's concept (1968) of simultaneous and relatively proportional increase of the severity of negative and positive symptoms in schizophrenia. However, in spite of the general tendency to simultaneous progression outlined earlier, either positive or negative symptoms could predominate at different time points of active disease period, and may show considerable fluctuations. Thus, the synchronization (or desynchronization, see later in this chapter) could be relative. And even at the stabilization stage of schizophrenia, positive symptoms still remain and constitute residual deficit states in a mixture with negative symptoms.

3.2.2 Relatively desynchronized trajectory of negative and positive symptoms

The desynchronized trajectory type presents with a long-term course of positive/negative symptoms that have bidirectional development vectors (see Fig. 3.2—diagrams II and III). In this case, there are two variants of the disease course with either negative or positive symptom progression. Negative schizophrenia (see Fig. 3.2—diagram II) and schizophrenia with negative symptoms that stopped at the very beginning of the disease (Smulevich, et al. 2017b Smulevich, et al. 2017) represent the forms of negative symptom progression (see Fig. 3.2).

Negative schizophrenia includes Bleuer's fundamental symptoms, or Huber's basic disturbances, or Carpenter's deficit syndrome determining the clinical presentation of the disease, and may progress over the course of schizophrenia with minimal severity (and tendency to further reduction) of positive symptoms as mild catatonic/paranoid symptoms observed mainly at the initial stage of the process.

In the so-called schizophrenia with negative symptoms that stopped at the very beginning (Smulevich, et al. 2017a; 2017b), negative symptoms, which are present at the initial stage (juvenile/adolescent period) of schizophrenia and have a strong association with personality traits/dimensions, show no or minimal further progression through the disease course after their initial onset. However, the further trajectory of the disease is characterized by positive symptoms.

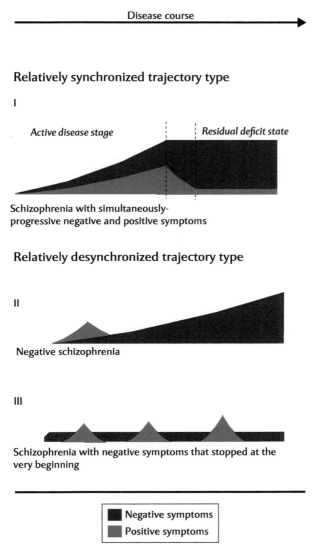

Figure 3.2 The model of two types of long-term course of primary negative symptoms in relation to positive symptoms: relatively synchronized or simultaneously progressive trajectory type (diagram I) versus relatively desynchronized or independently progressive trajectory type (diagrams II and III).

3.3 The concept of 'mutual/common syndromes' covers negative symptoms and personality/positive dimensions

The psychopathological model of 'mutual/common syndromes' represents a construct that describes the constellation of primary negative symptoms and personality/positive phenomena which are hybridized in unified clinical syndromes (Smulevich, et al. 2018; 2019). According to this model, primary negative symptoms, dichotomized on a dimensional basis (Galderisi, et al. 2013), constitute 'protopsychopathological entities'[2] that do not exist in 'a pure form' but only in association with personality traits and/or positive symptoms and/or general psychopathology features. Thus, in a clinical realm, primary negative symptoms in schizophrenia could be observed as *mixture states*,[3] resulting in a range of 'mutual/common syndromes'. As will be shown shortly, 'mutual/common syndromes' can be identified both in relatively synchronized and in relatively desynchronized trajectory types of the disease course. These *mixture syndromes* may appear during the course of schizophrenia at different time points: at the initial stage or as outcomes at the late stage (residual deficit states). The mutual/common syndromes depict the idea that negative symptoms in schizophrenia do not exist per se but interact with other clinical symptoms/features in particular ways which results in various phenotypical presentations during the disease course.

The description of common (*mixture*) syndromes may help in a better understanding and recognition of negative symptoms as parts of complex psychopathological structures.

3.4 Clinical characteristics of 'mutual/common syndromes'

This section includes a description of 'mutual/common syndromes' ('*mixture syndromes*') at the initial stage, and at the stabilization stage (residual deficit states), when negative/deficit symptoms of schizophrenia are clearly detectable.

The 'mutual/common syndromes' can be ranked according to the dichotomy of basic deficit or primary negative symptoms, that is, predominance of emotional (diminished expression) or motivational deficit (avolition).

---

[2] Since the biological nature of these disturbances is not fully understood, psychological and psychometric characteristics are mostly used to define them. Historically, these hypothetic pure deficit phenomena correspond to the fundamental symptoms of Bleuler.

[3] The term 'mixed' states is used in relation to bipolar disorders, and in order to avoid confusion, the term 'mixture' states has been used in this chapter in relation to schizophrenia.

3.5 The 'mutual/common syndromes' at the initial stage of schizophrenia

At the initial stage of schizophrenia, negative symptoms of 'mutual/common syndromes' are associated with personality dimensions and could resemble some intensified/amplified schizoid personality traits. These polarized traits (defensive or expansive) acquire dominant positions in the structure of 'mutual/common syndrome', being amplified by the corresponding underlying negative symptoms (avolition or diminished expression) (Smulevich, et al. 2018).

Accordingly, two corresponding types of initial stage 'mutual/common syndromes' could be distinguished: *the syndrome of defensive schizoid traits* with symptoms of volitional deficiency (avolition) and *the syndrome of expansive schizoid traits* with symptoms of diminished emotional expression.

3.5.1 The syndrome of defensive schizoid traits with symptoms of volitional deficiency (avolition)

This syndrome includes personality dimensions, characterized by passivity with 'discoloration' of personality traits and autistic escape from reality that manifests in the limited scope of communication and interpersonal contacts.

Avolition, as a predominant negative symptom, includes indecision, passivity, lack of initiative, obeying and symbiotic dependence on caregivers, and adherence to stereotypes with limited ability or inability to make independent decisions. Motivational disturbances are associated with the phenomena of reduction of the psychic energetic potential (anergy, passivity) and reduction or loss of spontaneous activity such as educational/occupational and other activities.

3.5.2 The syndrome of expansive schizoid traits with symptoms of diminished emotional expression (blunted affect)

The syndrome is determined by the oddity dimension that includes eccentricity, peculiarity of appearance and speech, and outspokenness as a deficiency in the understanding of the figurative sense of words and subtlety of metaphors. E. Kretschmer (1929) described 'loss of allopsychic resonance' with behavioural symptoms (loss of decorum and the ability to set personal boundaries) and change in lifestyle with nonconformity to social norms (autism with detachment from current social paradigm). Autistic activity may be observed in behaviour which includes eccentric, over-valued hobbies and the lack of long-term perspectives leading to professional instability and frequent changes in types of employment.

The phenomena of emotional deficiency include coldness; emotional paradoxicality, i.e. detachment from immediate relatives conjoined with irrational attachment to scatty persons; pragmatism ('pathological rationalism' or *rationalisme morbide*, according to E. Minkowski (1927)); establishment of interpersonal relations lacking empathy, emotional syntony ('co-sounding'), and social sensitivity.

3.6 The 'mutual/common syndromes' at the late stage of disease

At the stage of disease stabilization, negative symptoms, as part of corresponding 'mutual/common syndromes', may be combined with residual paranoid, catatonic, obsessive-compulsive, hallucinatory, and delusional symptoms (which constitute the residual deficit states of schizophrenia).

In residual deficit states, observed after long-term active continuous course of schizophrenia or after a series of episodes and 'shifts', negative symptoms are combined with reduced ('personalized') positive symptoms (e.g. mild paranoid and catatonic symptoms, the latter include dyskinetic movements, rituals, etc.) reflecting the respective symptomatology of a former active stage of schizophrenia (delusions, catatonia, obsessive-compulsive symptoms, etc.). Thus, schizophrenia residual states include deficits with (1) post-psychotic positive symptoms, or with (2) pseudo-neurotic symptoms.

3.6.1 Schizophrenia residual states with post-psychotic symptoms

'Hypoparanoid' syndrome with 'a new life' phenomenon
(W. Mayer-Gross, 1920) and symptoms of diminished emotional expression

This syndrome defines the clinical picture at the residual stage after long-term delusional psychosis. Symptoms of pronounced emotional deficiency are accompanied by a complete change in the individual's self-consciousness—alienation from former family, break with former friendships and social relations.

The hypoparanoid (over-valued) belief system, remaining after the intensity of delusions decrease, is associated with the abandonment of former personal values such as family relationships, profession, and religious beliefs. At the same time, the development of the concept of a 'new' life can be observed, which is autistic, with a separation from previous habits and attachments, an existence that is built not on the basis of past life experience (before the onset of schizophrenia) but under the influence of paranoid ideas which emerged during the period of psychosis.

Syndrome of 'dyskinetopathy' with symptoms of volitional deficiency

The syndrome represents a complex of motor residual symptoms after catatonic psychosis.

Among the negative dimensions, diminished initiative and intellectual activity, passivity, and a lack of independent, self-motivated decisions are in the foreground. The scope of activities is limited, and the general way of life is narrowed to a routine, not requiring alternative approaches or actions.

In the process of the formation of the residual state, there is a retention of rudimentary positive catatonic symptoms corresponding to the negative changes that have occurred. Stereotypies and perseverations are incorporated into the acquired 'mutual/common syndrome' pattern and support monotonous daily life activity. All types of everyday activities acquire a 'perseverative' automatic character implemented in the performance of a narrowly defined range of procedures, consisting mainly of elementary operations. The general way of life, including work and social activities, leisure, and daily routine such as a travel pattern around the city, the daily schedule, and dressing are subjected to established stereotypes.

3.6.2 Schizophrenia residual states with pseudo-neurotic features

Schizophrenic residual states with pseudo-neurotic features also correspond to the dichotomy of primary negative symptoms. The 'mutual/common syndromes' of schizoasthenia or schizophrenic asthenia (Ey, 1952; Sass and Parnas, 2003) and ritualized obsessions can be distinguished. Respectively, they are associated with the negative phenomena of volitional deficiency or diminished emotional expression.

3.6.2.1 Schizoasthenia syndrome with symptoms of volitional deficiency

The phenomenon of schizoasthenia, as a kind of schizophrenic residual state (Conrad, 1958; Glatzel, 1972), is observed after the long-term course of schizophrenia with the predominance of negative symptoms.

The dysfunctions of motivation (avolition) include lack of drive, diminished or even loss of spontaneous (without external stimulation) actions and reactions, difficulties with overcoming inertia, all of which interfere with activities in work and social life.

The loss of self-confidence, ambivalence, lack of endurance in achieving goals, abandonment of all types of activities, including employment, that require initiative, persistence, and permanent effort are in the foreground among the deficit symptoms.

Anergia, in schizoasthenia syndrome, is closely related to negative symptoms of avolition type and actually represents a marker of the underlying schizophrenic deficit (Smulevich, et al. 2019).

Accordingly, complaints of fatigue, a feeling of permanent tiredness (rest does not build up vigour and former capabilities), general unwellness, lack of strength, or even a feeling of sheer exhaustion dominate in the clinical picture of schizoasthenia. Along with subjective complaints, there is a pseudoneurasthenic symptomatology (exaggerated hyperesthesia, insomnia, signs of somatic malady, nausea, palpitations, headaches, faintness, etc.) which is not related to the exposure of exogenous hazards.

The reduction of the energetic potential, a decline in mental and physical activity and productivity resulting in deterioration in educational and professional achievements and episodes of attention and thought disturbances (concentration difficulties, loss of purposefulness, derailment, etc.) are among the core symptoms of schizoasthenia associated with a volitional deficiency.

There is a clear tendency to self-sparing behaviour—'energy saving', avoidance of physical and emotional efforts, limitation of interpersonal communication—described by Snezhnevsky (1968) as asthenic autism.

3.6.2.2 Syndrome of ritualized obsessions

The syndrome is formed on the termination of the active stage of schizophrenia proceeding with obsessions; schizo-obsessive subtype of schizophrenia (Zohar, 1997) or malignant obsessive-compulsive disorder. This syndrome is characterized by negative symptoms with a predominance of emotional deficiency (egocentrism with deficiency in empathy, pettiness, meanness, avarice, inflexibility, refusal to compromise).

At the stable stage, negative symptoms are associated with personalized obsessive-compulsive phenomena. Personalized obsessions typically relate to order or symmetry and behaviour resembling hording.

Ritualized obsessions are accompanied with exploitative behaviour and sadistic tendencies towards close relatives. Relatives are forcibly involved into participation and implementation of rituals. Also, the syndrome is characterized by rough manipulation of others, manifesting in explosive response reactions to the refusal to satisfy the sufferer's requirements. In accordance with the established schedule, patients devise a kind of 'home tyranny', with the involvement of relatives in a complex system of ritualized actions.

3.7 Implication for treatment

The treatment of negative symptoms associated with positive symptoms is beyond the scope of this chapter; see Chapters 5 and 6, which address the pharmacological and psychosocial treatments of negative symptoms.

The approach based on the concept of mutual/common syndromes offered earlier makes it possible to clarify the indications for psychopharmacotherapy beyond antipsychotics. Taking into account the positive symptoms associated with negative ones in the structure of mutual/common syndromes, it is justifiable to use combined treatment strategies. With this approach, targeting positive symptoms (hypoparanoic, pseudoasthenic, compulsive, etc.) closely associated with negative ones, the correction of complementary and potentially reversible subdomains of negative symptoms could be reached.

3.8 Conclusion

Negative symptoms in schizophrenia should be diagnosed and treated in consideration with a set of possible subtypes of their relationship with positive symptoms. The long-term course of negative symptoms should be evaluated both retrospectively and prospectively in addition to their cross-sectional evaluation (i.e. at a single point of time). The recognition of mutual/common syndromes in addition to individual negative symptoms may help in improving the diagnoses of negative/deficit schizophrenia with primary negative symptoms.

REFERENCES

Andreasen, N., Olsen, S. (1982). Negative vs positive schizophrenia. Definition and validation. *Archives of General Psychiatry.* **39**, 789–94.

Berze, J. (1914). *Die Primäre Insuffizienz der Psychischen Aktivität.* [The primary insufficiency of mental activity]: *ihr Wesen, ihre Erscheinungen und ihre Bedeutung als Grundstörung der Dementia Praecox und der Hypophrenien überhaupt.* Leipzig, Franz Deuticke.

Bleuler, E. (1911). *Dementia Praecox oder Gruppe der Schizophrenien.* Leipzig, Deuticke.

Carpenter, W., Heinrichs, D., Wagman, A. (1988). Deficit and nondeficit forms of schizophrenia: the concept. *American Journal of Psychiatry*, **145**(5), 578–83.

Conrad, K. (1958). *Die beginnende Schizophrenie.* Stuttgart, Georg Thieme.

Crow, T. J. (1980). Positive and negative schizophrenic symptoms and the role of dopamine. *British Journal of Psychiatry*, **151**, 199–204.

Delamillieure, P., Fernandez, J., Constans, J. M., Brazo, P., Benali, K., Abadie, P., et al. (2000). Proton magnetic resonance spectroscopy of the medial prefrontal cortex in patients with deficit schizophrenia: preliminary report. *American Journal of Psychiatry*, **157**(4), 641–3.

Delamillieure, P., Constans, J. M., Fernandez, J., Brazo, P., Dollfus, S. (2004). Relationship between performance on the Stroop test and N-acetylaspartate in the medial prefrontal cortex in deficit and nondeficit schizophrenia: preliminary result. *Psychiatry Research: Neuroimaging*, **132**, 87–9.

Ey, H. (1952). *Études psychiatriques.* Paris, Descleé de Brouwer.

Galderisi, S., Bucci, P., Mucci, A., Kirkpatrick, B., Pini, S., Rossi A., et al. (2013). Categorical and dimensional approaches to negative symptoms of schizophrenia: focus on long-term stability and functional outcome. *Schizophrenia Research*, **147**(1), 157–62.

Glatzel, J. (1972). Autochtone Asthenien. *Fortschritte der Neurologie-Psychiatrie*, **8**, 596–619

Huber, G. (1961). *Chronische Schizophrenie. Synopsis klinischer und neuroradiologischer Untersuchungen an defektschizophrenen Anstaltspatienten. Einzeldarstellungen aus der theoretischen und Klinischen Medizin.* Heidelberg, Dr. Huthig.

Huber, G. (1966). Reine defektsyndrome und Basisstadien endogener Psychosen. [Pure deficit syndromes and basic stages of endogenous psychoses.] *Fortschritte der Neurologie-Psychiatrie*, **34**, 409–26.

Huber, G. (1995). Prodrome der Schizophrenie. [Prodromal symptoms in schizophrenia]. *Fortschritte der Neurologie-Psychiatrie*, **63**(4), 131–8.

Jackson, J.H. (1889). On post-epileptic states: a contribution to the comparative study of insanities. British Journal of Psychiatry, 34(148), 490–500.

Kirschner, M., Aleman, A., Kaiser, S. (2017). Secondary negative symptoms—a review of mechanisms, assessment and treatment. *Schizophrenia Research*, **186**, 29–38.

Kraepelin, E. (1915). *Psychiatrie: Ein Lehrbuch für Studierende und Ärzte.* **8.**, volst. umgearb. Aufl. Leipzig, Johann Ambrosius Barth

Kretschmer, E. (1929). *Körperbau und Charakter.* Berlin, Verlag von Julius Springer.

Mayer-Gross, W. (1920). Über die Stellungnehme zur abgelaufenen akuten Psychose. Eine Studie über verständliche Zuzammenhänge in der Schizophrenie. *Zeitschrift für die gesamte Neurologie und Psychiatrie*, **60**, 160–213.

Minkowski, E. (1927). *La schizophrénie. Psychopathologie des schizoides et des schizophrènes*. Paris, Payot.

Mosolov, S. N., Potapov, A. V., Ushakov, U. V., Shafarenko, A. A., Kostyukova, A. B. (2014). Design and validation of standardized clinical and functional remission criteria in schizophrenia. *Neuropsychiatric Disease and Treatment*, **10**, 167–81.

Mucci, A., Merlotti E., Üçok, A., Aleman, A., Galderisi, S. (2017). Primary and persistent negative symptoms: concepts, assessments and neurobiological bases. *Schizophrenia Research*, Aug(186), 19–28.

Nkam, I., Thibaut, F., Denise, P., Van Der Elst, A., Ségard, L., Brazo, P., et al. (2001). Saccadic and smooth-pursuit eye movements in deficit and non deficit schizophrenia. *Schizophrenia Research*, **48**, 145–53.

Sass, H. (1989). The historical evolution of the concept of negative symptoms in schizophrenia. *British Journal of Psychiatry Supplement*, **7**, 26–31; discussion 37–40.

Sass, L. A., Parnas, J. (2003). Schizophrenia, consciousness, and the self. *Schizophrenia Bulletin*, **29**(3), 427–44.

Smulevich, A. B. (2016). Schizophrenia spectrum disorders in general medical practice. *Zhurnal Nevrologii i Psikhiatrii imeni S.S. Korsakova*, **116**(1), 4–9. (in Russian).

Smulevich, A. B., Romanov, D. V., Mukhorina, A. K, Atadzhikova, J. A. (2017a). 'Verschrobene'—phenomenon in schizophrenia and schizophrenia spectrum disorders: aspects of systematics. *Zhurnal Nevrologii i Psikhiatrii imeni S.S. Korsakova*, **117**(1), 5–16. (in Russian).

Smulevich, A. B., Romanov, D. V., Voronova, E. I., Mukhorina, A. K., Chitlova, V. V., Sorokina, O. Y. (2017b). Evolution of the schizophrenic deficit concept. *Zhurnal Nevrologii i Psikhiatrii imeni S.S. Korsakova*, **117**(9), 4–14. (in Russsian).

Smulevich, A. B., Dubnitskaya, E. B., Lobanova, V. M., Voronova, E. I., Zhylin, V. O., Kolyutskaya, E. V., et al. (2018). Personality disorders and schizophrenic defect (problem of comorbidity). *Zhurnal Nevrologii i Psikhiatrii imeni S.S. Korsakova*, **118**(11), 4–14. (in Russian).

Smulevich A. B., Kharkova G. S, Lobanova V. M., Voronova E. I. (2019) Asthenia in the psychopathological space of schizophrenia and schizophrenia spectrum disorders (the concept of the asthenic deficit in the modern model of negative symptoms' aspect) *Zhurnal Nevrologii i Psikhiatrii imeni S.S. Korsakova*, **119**(5), 7–14. (in Russian).

Snezhnevsky, A. V. (1968). 'The symptomatology, clinical forms and nosology of schizophrenia' in J. D. Howells (ed.), *Modern Perspectives in World Psychiatry*. Edinburgh, Oliver & Boyd, Ltd. pp. 425–447.

Trimble, M. R. (1986). Positive and negative symptoms in psychiatry. *British Journal of Psychiatry*, **148**, 587–9.

Voineskos, A. N., Foussias, G., Lerch, J., Felsky, D., Remington, G., Rajji, T. K., et al. (2013). Neuroimaging evidence for the deficit subtype of schizophrenia. *JAMA Psychiatry*, **70**, 472–80.

Zohar, J. (1997). Is there room for a new diagnostic subtype: the schizo-obsessive subtype? *CNS Spectrums*, **2**, 49–50.

CHAPTER 3

CHAPTER 4

The patients' view: Self-evaluation of negative symptoms

Sonia Dollfus and Anais Vandevelde

KEY POINTS

- The use and the choice of standardized assessment tools are necessary for improving identification of negative symptoms and for testing new, efficient therapies.
- Most of the scales on negative symptoms are based on observer rating. Compared to these scales, self-assessments have been overlooked. Nevertheless, they are quite relevant since they are generally simple; they allow the patients to report their own symptoms and so are complementary to the evaluations based on observer ratings; they require the patient's participation and so improve their involvement in the treatment; they are time-efficient and can be very useful for identification of negative symptoms at the onset of illness.
- Among the self-assessments, we can distinguish those designed and validated by researchers in groups of patients with schizophrenia and others that can be used in schizophrenia while they have been validated in other populations.
  - Among the first group, two recent scales have supplanted old scales, the Motivation and Pleasure Scale–Self-Report (MAP–SR) and the Self-evaluation of Negative Symptoms (SNS). The last presents all the psychometric properties required.
  - Among the second group, the most used scales are focused on anhedonia and apathy which assess these dimensions in schizophrenia but also in various psychiatric and neurological disorders; the most known are the Social Anhedonia Scale (SAS), the Physical Anhedonia Scale (PAS), and more recently are, on the one hand, the Self-reported Apathy Evaluation Scale (AES-S) and on the other, the Temporal Experience of Pleasure Scale (TEPS) and the Anticipatory and Consummatory Interpersonal Pleasure Scale (ACIPS), which distinguish anticipatory and consummatory pleasures.

4.1 Introduction

Negative symptoms are found in many patients with schizophrenia, and more so if we consider secondary negative symptoms to positive symptoms, substance use, medication side effects, or depression. Moreover, negative symptoms are responsible for impaired social functioning and quality of life, underlining the necessity to find efficient therapies targeting them. Compared to positive symptoms, negative symptoms have been overlooked in the diagnostic criteria, treatment, and even in clinical practice. This is probably due to the low efficacy of antipsychotics but also to the difficulty in assessing these symptoms. The first reason is the fact that negative symptoms overlap with other domains such as depression, and it is a real challenge to separate negative symptoms from depression in particular. Second, consensus on the identification and definition of negative symptoms is missing in Europe as a whole and even within a single country.

In this context, the section and use of standardized assessment tools are necessary across the European Union for improving identification of negative symptoms, testing new efficient therapies, and also for research to investigate the brain abnormalities underlying negative symptoms. Nevertheless, it is quite surprising to note that scales are underused in the evaluation of negative symptoms in schizophrenia compared to scales used in depression. Most of the scales on negative symptoms are based on observer rating or clinician's instrument. We identified 18 scales based on observer rating compared to only 5 self-reports from which only 2 can really be considered as self-assessments (Mach and Dollfus, 2016; Llerena, Park, McCarthy, et al. 2013); most of the observer-based rating scales are dimensional scales, and two recent scales are the Brief Negative Symptom Scales (BNSS; Kirkpatrick, Strauss, Nguyen, et al. 2011) and the Clinical Assessment Interview for Negative Symptoms (CAINS) (Kring, Gur Blanchard, et al. 2013). Only one is a categorical scale, the Schedule of Deficit Syndrome (SDS; Kirkpatrick, Buchanan, McKenny, et al. 1989) that can categorize patients into deficit and non-deficit subtypes. Compared to these scales based on observer ratings, self-assessments have been overlooked, probably because of the idea that patients with schizophrenia with negative symptoms are unable to report their own symptoms accurately (Hamera, Schneider, Potocky, et al. 1996; Selten, Wiersma, and Van Den Bosch, 2000).

In our opinion, the self-assessments are quite relevant. They are generally very simple, and self-reporting forms are easy for the patient to complete since they have simple questions, short sentences, and easy, multiple-choice answers, not more than three or four for each item. Self-evaluation allows the patients to report their overall functioning and their own symptoms; the patient is not influenced by the questions of the rater and so the resulting report is entirely subjective. These evaluations require patient participation and so improve their involvement in their own treatment. Moreover, self-assessment is time-efficient, taking less time than a clinician's evaluation; some self-reports only take 5 minutes while evaluations based on interview can take more than 20 minutes to complete. Self-evaluations are complementary to the evaluations based on observer ratings; they can provide clinical information not necessarily detected by caregivers or medical staff in a standard interview. In particular, self-assessments allow the patient to express their own feelings and a subjective level of awareness of their symptoms. Finally, self-assessments can be very useful for identifying negative symptoms at the onset of illness. Indeed, negative symptoms appear early, long before positive symptoms, have a high prevalence compared to attenuated positive symptoms, might go unnoticed and consequently untreated, leading to poorer functioning. Moreover, they have been reported to be predictive of transition to psychosis (Piskulic, Addington, Cadenhead, et al. 2012). It is again surprising that self-reports have been developed for evaluating psychotic symptoms in schizophrenia (Niv, Cohen, Mintz, et al. 2007) and prodromal psychotic symptoms (Kobayashi, Nemoto, Koshikawa, et al. 2008; Kelleher, Harley, Murtagh, et al. 2011) but not for screening negative symptoms.

Among the self-assessments, we can distinguish those focusing on the negative domains of schizophrenia, created by researchers and validated in patients with schizophrenia and those which can self-measure negative symptoms of schizophrenia but have been validated in other populations (healthy subjects, patients with personality or neurological disorders) and so may not be specific to schizophrenia.

4.1.1 Self-assessments of negative symptoms developed in schizophrenia

For self-assessments to be valid, they should have the same properties as the scales based on observer ratings on negative symptoms of schizophrenia. They should cover the five domains of negative symptoms (anhedonia, alogia, avolition, blunted affect, social withdrawal), present good convergent and divergent validities, display the five negative domains with factorial analysis, and measure the negative symptoms whatever the language and culture. Moreover, self-reports should be brief and easy to understand, present good intra-subject reliability, and have a well-defined threshold from which negative symptoms can be considered as pathological.

Historically, three scales were developed to assess subjective experience of deficit or negative symptoms.

The Subjective Deficit Syndrome Scale (SDSS) (Jaeger, Bitter, Czobor, et al. 1990) allows reporting patient complaints but this scale is not solely focused on negative symptoms and other complaints were not correlated with negative symptoms. It is viewed as a variant of Huber's pure defect syndrome, limited to subjective complaints. The advantage is that it is brief and can be completed in five to ten minutes (experience is rated in 'yes' or 'no' responses, distress and disturbance are rated according to four degrees). The disadvantage is that the scale contains 19 items and only 3 focus on negative symptoms. Other items are not negative symptoms (e.g. insomnia, coenesthetic experiences, and decreased patience).

The Subjective Experience of Deficits in Schizophrenia scale (SEDS) (Liddle and Barnes, 1988) was designed to measure subjective awareness of deficits on thought and mental activity. Again, only a few items evaluate the negative dimension and the ratings are made on the basis of a semi-standardized interview, not on a self-assessment.

The Subjective Experience of Negative Symptoms scale (SENS) (Selten, Sijben, Van Den Bosch, et al. 1993) was also devised on the basis of a semi-standardized interview, based on the latest version of the Scale of Assessment of Negative Symptoms (SANS) (Andreasen, 1989). SENS is an interview-based self-rating tool designed to measure several aspects of the subjective experience of negative symptoms, such as awareness, causal attribution, and disruption or distress. However, to our knowledge, neither convergent nor discriminant validity has been tested for this scale.

Recently, the Motivation and Pleasure Scale–Self-Report (MAP–SR) was developed (Llerena, Park, McCarthy, et al. 2013). It is a 15-item self-report version of the CAINS Motivation and Pleasure subscale. All items are rated on a five-point Likert scale. It is a short scale and has demonstrated good validity. Due to poor reliability and validity, the emotional expression (blunted affect and alogia) rating from the first version of the CAINS self-report (Park, Llerena, McCarthy, et al. 2012) was removed, giving rise to a revised measure that focuses exclusively on self-reported deficits in motivation and pleasure. Thus, the disadvantage is that this self-assessment only covers two negative domains (pleasure and motivation), and emotional expression is excluded. This point might be considered a weakness of the scale since emotional expression (from CAINS) might allow us to differentiate between negative and depressive symptoms (Richter, Holz, Hesse, et al. 2019). As a strong overlap of negative and depressive symptoms is observed (these symptoms notably concern avolition, social withdrawal, and anhedonia), identifying symptoms which can differentiate both domains is essential to adapt therapeutic strategies. Moreover, the evaluation contains many questions containing questions regarding 'how often' and 'how much', which require that patients remember and quantify what feelings or events happened in the past week, potentially difficult for patients with memory impairment.

That is why we developed Self-evaluation of Negative Symptoms (SNS) that offers the following characteristics:

1. SNS is very simple in design and content (Dollfus, Mach, and Morello, 2016). It contains 20 concise statements, easily understandable since they are verbatim from patients with schizophrenia. The number of responses was voluntarily limited to three in order to simplify completion and avoid random responses when score ranges are too broad. The patient has a choice of only three answers: 'Strongly agree', 'Somewhat agree', and 'Strongly disagree', with a corresponding score of 2, 1, and 0 respectively. The total score ranges from 0 (no negative symptoms) to 40 (severe negative symptoms).

2. The scale measures the five domains of negative symptoms (social withdrawal, emotional range, avolition, anhedonia, and alogia) as required and determined by the US consensus conference on negative symptoms (Kirkpatrick, Fenton, Carpenter, et al. 2006). The scale therefore

contains five subscores evaluated by four items. As the blunted affect (defined by reduced facial expression, vocal expression, and expressive gestures) is evaluated only on the behaviour in observed-based ratings, it was replaced by the emotional dimension called 'diminished emotional range' that evaluates the patients' capacity to express and feel emotions. For example, one of these items (item 6) is: 'There are many happy or sad things in life but I don't feel concerned by them'.

3. SNS presents good convergent and discriminant validities. In the first validation study including 49 patients with schizophrenia and schizoaffective disorders (Dollfus, et al. 2016), SNS was significantly correlated with the SANS ($r = 0.628$), supporting good convergent validity. SNS scores were not correlated with Parkinsonism ($r = 0.175$), or with Brief Psychiatric Rating Scale (BPRS) positive subscores ($r = 0.253$) in favour of good discriminant validity. The most interesting result was the absence of any correlation between the SNS scores and the insight scale (IS) (Birchwood, Smith, Drury, et al. 1994) scores ($r = -0.008$), demonstrating that patients with negative symptoms can evaluate their negative symptoms independently of their level of insight of illness, contrarily to what has been reported in the literature (Sevy, Nathanson, Visweswaraiah, et al. 2004; Saeedi, Addington, and Addington, 2007). Negative and depressive symptoms cannot be differentiated easily, since a strong overlap between both domains is expected. Notably, the avolition factor of negative symptoms encompasses symptoms that also belongs to the main symptoms of depression: loss of interest, anhedonia, and reduced energy. Moreover, up to 80 per cent of patients with schizophrenia experience an episode of major depression (Upthegrove, Birchwood, Ross, et al. 2010), underlining the frequent associations of depressive and negative symptoms in patients with schizophrenia. In our study, we found a significant correlation between the SNS and the Calgary Depression Scale for Schizophrenia (CDSS) (Addington, Addington, and Maticka-Tyndale, 1993) in 49 patients (Dollfus, Mach, Morello, 2016). However, the lack of a significant correlation between diminished emotional range of SNS and depressed mood (the first item of the CDSS) demonstrates that patients are able to distinguish loss of emotion from depressive mood. These results accord with those of Richer and colleagues (Richter, Holz, Hesse, et al. 2019) that showed that emotional expression from the CAINS can discriminate between subjects with depression and those with schizophrenia. Taken together, therefore, these results allow us to consider the reduction of felt emotion and the experienced depressed mood as two domains that might be more specific regarding negative symptoms on one hand and depression on the other hand in patients with schizophrenia and depressive symptoms.

4. A self-assessment scale needs to have a good reliability that means that patients with a stable clinical state must assess it in the same manner at

two distinct times. So, a second SNS was scheduled 4–8 weeks after the first one in 49 stable patients characterized by no increase in symptoms and no change in doses of psychotropic drugs or social therapy since the first assessment. The test-retest reliability was excellent (ICC = 0.942) demonstrating good stability of evaluations supporting the finding that patients with negative symptoms can self-assess correctly (Dollfus, Mach, Morello, 2016).

5. A factorial structure of the SNS was examined using a principal component analysis (PCA) with a varimax rotation in 245 patients coming from a European sample (Mucci, Vignapiano, Bitter, et al. 2019). The optimal number of factors was determined with an eigenvalue > 1.0 and screen plot criteria. The items with robust loadings > 0.42 after varimax rotation were used to interpret the extracted factors. We found five factors that matched with the five subscales of SNS (Table 4.1). Indeed, the four items from each subscale of SNS was loaded on the corresponding negative domains; only one item from the anhedonia subscale was loaded on the social withdrawal factor. So, the factorial structure of SNS supports the idea of five domains of negative symptoms in accordance with Strauss and colleagues (Strauss, Nunez, Ahmed, et al. 2018). These results are not contradictory with those observed with a factorial analysis on the five subscores of SNS that displayed two components, felt emotion and apathy. Indeed, these two components might be second-order factors while the five domains might be first-order factors, as Strauss and colleagues found with a hierarchical model on scales based on observer ratings (Strauss, Nunez, Ahmed, et al. 2018).

6. Sensitivity, specificity, and a threshold beyond which the negative symptoms are considered pathological were tested in a comparative study of 109 patients with schizophrenia or schizoaffective disorders (DSM-5) and 99 healthy subjects using the SNS (Dollfus, Delouche, Hervochon, et al. 2019). A receiver operating characteristic (ROC) curve was created by plotting the true positive rate (sensitivity) against the false positive rate (1– specificity) at various threshold settings. The best identified threshold was 7 with a sensitivity and specificity at 92.7 per cent (95% CI = 86.1 to 96.8) and 85.9% (95% CI = 77.4 to 92.1) respectively. This meant that 92.7 per cent of patients with schizophrenia had a score of SNS above 7, and 85.9 per cent of healthy subjects had a score of SNS under 7. These results indicate that SNS might be useful for screening negative symptoms in clinical practice. However, further studies using SNS in subjects at high risk for psychosis or with a first psychotic episode are needed.

7. Demonstrating that a scale can measure negative symptoms whatever the culture and language is another important characteristic of a scale. The first step is to translate the scale into several different languages. At this time, SNS is available in 16 languages with back translations validated

Table 4.1 Principal component analysis of SNS after varimax rotation

Negative dimension	The 20 items of SNS	Components				
		1	2	3	4	5
	SNS.14. It's hard to stick to doing things on an everyday regular basis	.806	.160	.122	.040	.040
	SNS.13. I find it difficult to meet the objectives I set myself	.708	.026	.044	.163	.080
AVOLITION	SNS.15. There are many things I don't do through lack of motivation or because I don't feel like it	.701	.095	.151	.352	.143
	SNS.16. I know there are things I must do (get up or wash myself, for example) but I have no energy	.677	.143	.130	.017	.174
	SNS.1. I prefer to be alone in my corner	.091	.796	.088	−.084	.094
SOCIAL WITHDRAWAL	SNS.2. I'm better off alone because I feel uncomfortable when anyone is near me	.319	.694	.127	−.016	.189
	SNS.3. I'm not interested in going out with friends or family	.096	.599	.095	.480	.129
	SNS.4. I don't particularly try to contact and meet friends (letters, telephone, text messaging, etc.)	.029	.560	.321	.342	.027
	SNS.17. I don't take any great pleasure in talking to people	.262	.420	.266	.282	.226
	SNS.11. People often say that I don't talk much	.026	.116	.762	−.035	.225
ALOGIA	SNS.10. I find it ten times harder to talk to than most people do	.241	.164	.733	.110	.072
	SNS.9. I don't have as much to talk about as most people	.103	.100	.615	.251	.282
	SNS.12. With friends and family, I want to talk about things but it doesn't come out	.409	.234	.438	.152	.077
	SNS.20. I am not interested in having sex	.051	−.068	.106	.714	.092
	SNS.18. I find it hard to take pleasure even when doing things I have chosen to do	.445	.227	.043	.619	.158

continued >

Table 4.1 Continued

Negative dimension	The 20 items of SNS	Components				
		1	2	3	4	5
ANHEDONIA	SNS.19. When I imagine doing one thing or another, I don't feel any particular pleasure in the idea	.340	.249	.146	.606	.198
EMOTIONAL FEELING	SNS.5. People say I'm not sad or happy and that I'm not often angry	.139	.108	.074	−.003	.699
	SNS.7. Watching a sad or happy film, reading, or listening to a sad or happy story does not especially make me want to cry or laugh	.059	−.031	.238	.208	.659
	SNS.6. There are many happy or sad things in life but I don't feel concerned by them	.023	.366	.047	.219	.629
	SNS.8. It is difficult for people to know how I feel	.183	.100	.204	.061	.574

according to the guidelines (Wild, Grove, Martin, et al. 2005). A study is underway in a sample constituted of 245 patients with schizophrenia coming from 10 European countries. The scales are available on request to dollfus-s@chu-caen.fr.

4.1.2 Self-assessments of negative symptoms developed in disorders other than schizophrenia

Negative symptoms are considered as core features in patients with psychotic disorders. Although traditionally described only in relation to schizophrenia, negative symptoms may also occur in other mental disorders such as schizophrenia-spectrum disorders, neurological disorders, and also in the general, 'non-clinical' population.

Most self-assessment scales of negative domains cannot discriminate negative symptoms between neuropsychiatric disorders. Some scales cover the negative symptoms of schizophrenia while others are used in non-psychotic disorders to assess anhedonia and avolition in particular. Most of these scales were not developed and validated for schizophrenia specifically (Lincoln, Dollfus, and Lyne, 2016) (Table 4.2).

4.1.2.1 Self-report of psychiatric experiences

The Community Assessment of Psychic Experiences (CAPE) (Stefanis, Hanssen, Simmis, et al. 2002) rates lifetime psychotic experiences in the general population. It includes 42 items that assess low-grade psychotic, negative, and depressive experiences. The negative symptom factor includes 14 items derived from the SANS and the SENS. The CAPE negative items loaded on to the factors asociality, amotivation, and anhedonia that are related with depression but not with the PANSS negative scale (Schlier, Jaya, Moritz, et al. 2015).

4.1.2.2 Anhedonia

Anhedonia is the most commonly reported negative symptom in non-psychotic psychiatric disorders. It was first documented by Ribot (1896) and is defined as the loss of capacity to experience pleasure. Since this original report, anhedonia has been identified as a symptom of several different mental disorders, including schizophrenia, depression, and autism, but also other psychiatric and neurocognitive disorders. Several scales have been designed to assess a patient's subjective experiences of anhedonia or hedonic capacity in schizophrenia but also in other psychiatric disorders (Chapman, Chapman, and Raulin, 1976; Eckblad, Chapman, Chapman, et al. 1982; Olivares and Berrios, 1998; Reise, Horan, and Blanchard, 2011). In the last 15 years, there has been a resurgence in refining anhedonia scales, with two new published self-report questionnaires used in schizophrenia and other psychiatric disorders both of which attempt to take into account different facets of reward function with the consummatory and anticipatory pleasures (Gard, King, Gard, et al. 2007; Goding and Pflum, 2014).

Table 4.2 Self-rating scales measuring negative dimensions in non-psychotic psychiatric disorders

Scale	Description	Population	Dimension
Revised Social Anhedonia Scale (SAS)	40-item true/false scale —assesses the ability to experience pleasure into various domains	Schizophrenia Autism Personality disorder Major depressive disorder Alcohol abuse Eating disorder Social anxiety Healthy controls	Social anhedonia
Revised Physical Anhedonia Scale (PAS)	61-item true/false scale —high scores indicate more severe physical anhedonia	Schizophrenia Major depressive disorder Bipolar disorder Alcohol abuse Parkinson disease Eating disorder Healthy controls	Physical anhedonia
Self-Assessment Anhedonia Scale (SAAS)	27 items and 3 domains per item (intensity, frequency, and change), 11-point scale for each of the 3 domains, distinguishes the different types of anhedonia, measures perception of change in the patient's hedonic capacity	Schizophrenia Major depressive disorder	Anhedonia
Temporal Experience of Pleasure Scale (TEPS)	18-item, 6-point scale ('very false for me' to 'very true for me', separate scale for anticipatory and consummatory reward	Healthy students Bipolar disorder	Anhedonia
Anticipatory and Consummatory Interpersonal Pleasure Scale (ACIPS)	17-item, 6-point scale, only measures social anhedonia	Schizophrenia Healthy controls	Social anhedonia
Self-report Apathy Evaluation Scale (AES-S)	18-item, 4-point scale, evaluates self-experienced motivation and interests during the previous 4 weeks, does not include measures of functioning	Schizophrenia Stroke Subarachnoid haemorrhage Parkinson disease Multiple sclerosis Alzheimer's disease	Avolition– apathy

4.1.2.2.1 The Social Anhedonia Scale (SAS)

The Social Anhedonia Scale (SAS) or the Revised Social Anhedonia Scale (R-SAS) (Eckblad, et al. 1982) is the most commonly used measure of social anhedonia. It assesses pleasure experienced when interacting with others and interest in having close social connections. Studies have demonstrated that higher scores on the SAS are associated with poorer psychological and social functioning, and with poorer prognosis among individuals with schizophrenia and depression (Blanchard, Collins, Aghevli, et al. 2011), and are predictive of onset of schizophrenia spectrum disorders (Kwapil, 1998; Blanchard, Collins, Aghevli, et al. 2011).

4.1.2.2.2 The Physical Anhedonia Scale (PAS)

The Physical Anhedonia Scale (PAS) (Chapman, Chapman, and Raulin, 1976) assesses the experiences of pleasure in response to physical stimuli (taste, sight, touch, and smell). It is a 61-item self-report questionnaire, requiring 'Yes/No' answers. Each question is scored at 0 or 1 and the total score ranges from 0 to 61. Higher scores on PAS indicate greater levels of PA. Physical anhedonia has been studied as a marker of vulnerability to schizophrenia and endogenous depressions (Katsanis, Iacono, Beiser, et al. 1992; Loas, Dhee-Perot, Chaperot, et al. 1998).

SAS, R-SAS, and PAS are widely used to assess anhedonia in non-psychotic psychiatric disorders. Studies exploring social and physical anhedonia used these scales in major depression (Pelizza and Ferrari, 2009), social phobia (Meyer and Lenzenweger, 2009), eating disorders (Deborde, Berthoz, Godart, et al. 2006), autism spectrum disorders (Carre, Chevalier, Robel, et al. 2015), alcoholism (Marra, Warot, Payan, et al. 2998), and Parkinson's disease (Isella, Iurlaro, Piolti, et al. 2003). PAS and SAS do not discriminate anhedonia between patients with different psychiatric disorders. To correct this limit, the SAS was revised in order to discriminate social anhedonia from social anxiety (Cicero, Krieg, Becker, et al. 2016). However, some authors have found that SAS and R-SAS correlated with DSM-III personality disorder type A (paranoid, schizoid, and schizotypal personality disorders) and that such correlation dissolved in relatives of schizophrenic patients (Thaker, Moran, Adam, et al. 1993). Others have reported an association between high PAS scores and premorbid state in non-schizophrenic psychiatric inpatients (Garnet, Glick, and Edell, 1993).

4.1.2.2.3 The Self-Assessment Anhedonia Scale (SAAS)

As the PAS and R-SAS failed to distinguish the different types of anhedonia and to measure the perception of change in the patient's hedonic capacity, SAAS was designed to measure subjective change in the capacity to experience pleasure and to discriminate anhedonia between psychiatric disorders (Olivares, Berrios, and Bousono, 2005). The Self-Assessment Anhedonia Scale (SAAS) is based on a model that 'anhedonia' is a final common pathway onto which converge phenomena formed by different mechanisms (i.e. the so-called anhedonia of schizophrenia would be a different phenomenon from the 'true anhedonia' of depression) (Olivares and Berrios, 1998).

4.1.2.2.4 The Temporal Experience of Pleasure Scale (TEPS)

The Temporal Experience of Pleasure Scale (TEPS) has 18 items with two subscales designed to distinguish anticipatory and consummatory pleasures (Gard, Kring, Gard, et al. 2007). The scale takes 5-10 minutes to be filled. Items only reflect physical anhedonia. The scale was validated in a student population and was extended to schizophrenia and bipolar disorder populations (Tso, Grove, and Taylor, 2014). A significant advantage of this scale is that its two-factor structure separates anticipatory and consummatory pleasures.

4.1.2.2.5 The Anticipatory and Consummatory Interpersonal Pleasure Scale (ACIPS)

The Anticipatory and Consummatory Interpersonal Pleasure Scale (ACIPS) is a 17-item self-report that focuses on anhedonia related to social interactions and takes approximatively five to ten minutes to complete (Goodig and Pflum, 2014). The focus on social anhedonia is derived from research reporting that a high level of social anhedonia might be a risk factor for schizophrenia-spectrum disorders. The ACIPS was constructed to distinguish anticipation and consummatory pleasures.

4.1.2.3 Apathy

Negative symptoms also occur in several DSM-5 neurocognitive disorders and are commonly referred as apathy in this context. The Apathy Evaluation Scale is commonly used to evaluate neurological disorders such as Parkinson disease, Alzheimer's disease, multiple sclerosis, and stroke but also apathy in schizophrenia. This rating scale highlighted the high prevalence of apathy in the neurological diseases (Table 4.2) (Foussias, Agid, Fervaha, et al. 2014).

4.1.2.3.1 The Apathy Evaluation Scale Self-reported (AES-S)

Recently, Faerden and colleagues (Faerden, Lyngstad, Simonsen, et al. 2018) validated a shortened Apathy Evaluation Scale Self-reported (AES-S). It is a 12-item scale, each item scoring on a 4-point Likert scale. This version was taking out the same six items as in the shortened AES-Clinical rated. Higher scores indicate severe apathy. The questions focus on the degree of self-experienced motivation and interests during the last four weeks and do not include measures of functioning.

4.2 Conclusion

Among the rating scales, self-reported scales are particularly relevant since they assess subjective aspects of negative symptoms. They provide a measure of the patient's perception of his/her own symptoms, which is not possible with observer ratings. Self-rating scales are designed for frequent use. Consequently, they can save clinicians' and researchers' time by rapidly identifying patients with relevant subjective complaints related to the negative symptoms.

REFERENCES

Addington, D., Addington, J., Maticka-Tyndale, E. (1993). Assessing depression in schizophrenia: the Calgary Depression Scale. *British Journal of Psychiatry*, **163**(suppl 22), 39–44.

Andreasen, N. C. (1989). The scale for the assessment of negative symptoms (SANS): conceptual and theoretical foundations. *British Journal of Psychiatry*, **155**(suppl 7), 53–8.

Birchwood, M., Smith, J., Drury, V., Healy, J., MacMillan, F., Slade, M. (1994). A self-report Insight Scale for psychosis: reliability, validity and sensitivity to change. *Acta Psychiatrica Scandinavica*, **89**(1), 62–7.

Blanchard, J. J., Collins, L. M., Aghevli, M., Leung, W. W., Cohen, A. S. (2011). Social anhedonia and schizotypy in a community sample: the Maryland longitudinal study of schizotypy. *Schizophrenia Bulletin*, **37**(3), 587–602.

Carre, A., Chevallier, C., Robel, L., Barry, C., Maria, A. S., Pouga, L., et al. (2015). Tracking social motivation systems deficits: the affective neuroscience view of autism. *Journal of Autism Development Disorders*, **45**(10), 3351–63.

Chapman, L. J., Chapman, J. P., Raulin, M. L. (1976). Scales for physical and social anhedonia. *Journal of Abnormal Psychology*, **85**(4), 374–82.

Cicero, D. C., Krieg, A., Becker, T. M., Kerns, J. G. (2016). Evidence for the discriminant validity of the revised social anhedonia scale from social anxiety. *Assessment*, **23**(5), 544–56.

Deborde, A.S., Berthoz, S., Godart, N., Perdereau, F., Corcos, M., Jeammet, P. (2006). [Relations between alexithymia and anhedonia: a study in eating disordered and control subjects]. *Encephale*, **32**(1 Pt 1), 83–91.

Dollfus, S., Delouche, C., Hervochon, C., Mach, C., Bourgeois, V., Rotharmel, M., et al. (2019). Specificity and sensitivity of the self-assessment of negative symptoms in patients with schizophrenia. *Schizophrenia Research*, 2019. 211, 51–5.

Dollfus, S., Mach, C., Morello, R. (2016). Self-evaluation of negative symptoms: a novel tool to assess negative symptoms. *Schizophrenia Bulletin*, **42**(3), 571–8.

Eckblad, M. L., Chapman, L. J., Chapman, J. P., Mishlove, M. (1982). *The Revised Social Anhedonia Scale*. Unpublished test, University of Wisconsin, Madison.

Faerden, A., Lyngstad, S. H., Simonsen, C., Ringen, P. A., Papsuev, O., Dieset, I., et al. (2018). Reliability and validity of the self-report version of the apathy evaluation scale in first-episode Psychosis: concordance with the clinical version at baseline and 12 months follow-up. *Psychiatry Research*, **267**, 140–7.

Foussias, G., Agid, O., Fervaha, G., Remington, G. (2014). Negative symptoms of schizophrenia: clinical features, relevance to real world functioning and specificity versus other CNS disorders. *European Neuropsychopharmacology*, **24**(5), 693–709.

Gard, D. E., Kring, A. M., Gard, M. G., Horan, W. P., Green, M. F. (2007). Anhedonia in schizophrenia: distinctions between anticipatory and consummatory pleasure. *Schizophrenia Research*, **93**(1–3), 253–60.

Garnet, K. E., Glick, M., Edell, W. S. (1993). Anhedonia and premorbid competence in young, nonpsychotic psychiatric inpatients. *Journal of Abnormal Psychology*, **102**(4), 580–3.

Gooding, D. C., Pflum, M. J. (2014). The assessment of interpersonal pleasure: introduction of the Anticipatory and Consummatory Interpersonal Pleasure Scale (ACIPS) and preliminary findings. *Psychiatry Research*, **215**(1), 237–43.

Hamera, E. K., Schneider, J. K., Potocky, M., Casebeer, M. A. (1996). Validity of self-administered symptom scales in clients with schizophrenia and schizoaffective disorders. *Schizophrenia Research*, **19**(2–3), 213–19.

Isella, V., Iurlaro, S., Piolti, R., Ferrarese, C,. Frattola, L., Appollonio, I., et al. (2003). Physical anhedonia in Parkinson's disease. *Journal of Neurology, Neurosurgery and Psychiatry*, **74**(9), 1308–11.

Jaeger, J., Bitter, I., Czobor, P., Volavka, J. (1990). The measurement of subjective experience in schizophrenia: the subjective deficit syndrome scale. *Comprehensive Psychiatry*, **31**(3), 216–26.

Katsanis, J., Iacono, W. G., Beiser, M., Lacey, L. (1992). Clinical correlates of anhedonia and perceptual aberration in first-episode patients with schizophrenia and affective disorder. *Journal of Abnormal Psychology*, **101**(1), 184–91.

Kelleher, I., Harley, M., Murtagh, A., Cannon, M. (2011). Are screening instruments valid for psychotic-like experiences? A validation study of screening questions for psychotic-like experiences using in-depth clinical interview. *Schizophrenia Bulletin*, **37**(2), 362–9.

Kirkpatrick, B., Strauss, G., Nguyen, L., Fischer, B. A., Daniel, D. G., Cienfuegos, A., et al. (2011). The brief negative symptom scale: psychometric properties. *Schizophrenia Bulletin*, **37**(2).

Kirkpatrick, B., Fenton, W. S., Carpenter, W. T., Jr., Marder, S. R. (2006). The NIMH-MATRICS consensus statement on negative symptoms. *Schizophrenia Bulletin*, **32**(2), 214–19.

Kirkpatrick, B., Buchanan, R. W., McKenny, P. D., Alphs, L. D., Carpenter, W. T., Jr., (1989). The schedule for the deficit syndrome: an instrument for research in schizophrenia. *Psychiatry Research*, **30**, 119–23.

Kobayashi, H., Nemoto, T., Koshikawa, H., Osono, Y., Yamazawa, R., Murakami, M., et al. (2008). A self-reported instrument for prodromal symptoms of psychosis: testing the clinical validity of the PRIME Screen-Revised (PS-R) in a Japanese population. *Schizophrenia Research*, **106**(2–3), 356–62.

Kring, A. M., Gur, R. E., Blanchard, J. J., Horan, W. P., Reise, S. P. (2013). The Clinical Assessment Interview for Negative Symptoms (CAINS): final development and validation. *American Journal of Psychiatry*, **170**(2), 165–72.

Kwapil, T. R. (1998). Social anhedonia as a predictor of the development of schizophrenia-spectrum disorders. *Journal of Abnormal Psychology*, **107**(4), 558–65.

Liddle, P. F., Barnes, T. R. (1988). The subjective experience of deficits in schizophrenia. *Comprehensive Psychiatry*, **29**(2), 157–64.

Lincoln, T. M., Dollfus, S., Lyne, J. (2016). Current developments and challenges in the assessment of negative symptoms. *Schizophrenia Research*, **186**, 8–18.

Llerena, K., Park, S. G., McCarthy, J. M., Couture, S. M., Bennett, M. E., Blanchard, J. J. (2013). The Motivation and Pleasure Scale–Self-Report (MAP–SR): reliability and validity of a self-report measure of negative symptoms. *Comprehensive Psychiatry*, **54**(5), 568–74.

Loas, G., Dhee-Perot, P., Chaperot, C., Fremaux, D., Gayant, C., Boyer, P. (1998). Anhedonia, alexithymia and locus of control in unipolar major depressive disorders. *Psychopathology*, **31**(4), 206–12.

Mach, C., Dollfus, S. (2016). [Scale for assessing negative symptoms in schizophrenia: A systematic review]. *Encephale*, April, **42**(2), 165–71.

Marra, D., Warot, D., Payan, C., Hispard, E., Dally, S., Puech, A, J. (1998). Anhedonia and relapse in alcoholism. *Psychiatry Research*, **80**(2), 187–96.

Meyer, E. C., Lenzenweger, M. F. (2009). The specificity of referential thinking: a comparison of schizotypy and social anxiety. *Psychiatry Research*, **165**(1–2), 78–87.

Mucci, A., Vignapiano, A., Bitter, I., Austin, S. F., Delouche, C., Dollfus, S., et al. (2019). A large European, multicenter, multinational validation study of the brief negative symptom scale. *Neuropsychopharmacology*, August, **29**(8), 947–59.

Niv, N., Cohen, A. N., Mintz, J., Ventura, J., Young, A. S. (2007). The validity of using patient self-report to assess psychotic symptoms in schizophrenia. *Schizophrenia Research*, **90**(1–3), 245–50.

Olivares, J. M., Berrios, G. E. (1998). The anhedonias: clinical and neurobiological aspects. *International Journal of Psychiatry in Clinical Practice*, 2(3), 157–71.

Olivares, J. M., Berrios, G. E., Bousono, M. (2005). The self-assessment anhedonia scale. *Neurology, Psychiatry, and Brain Research*, **12**(3), 121–34.

Park, S. G., Llerena, K., McCarthy, J. M., Couture, S. M., Bennett, M. E., Blanchard, J. J. (2012). Screening for negative symptoms: preliminary results from the self-report version of the Clinical Assessment Interview for Negative Symptoms. *Schizophrenia Bulletin*, **135**(1–3), 139–43.

Pelizza, L., Ferrari, A. (2009). Anhedonia in schizophrenia and major depression: state or trait? *Annals in General Psychiatry*, **8**, 22.

Piskulic, D., Addington, J., Cadenhead, K. S., Cannon, T. D., Cornblatt, B. A., Heinssen, R., et al. (2012). Negative symptoms in individuals at clinical high risk of psychosis. *Psychiatry Research*, **196**(2–3), 220–4.

Reise, S. P., Horan, W. P., Blanchard, J. J. (2011). The challenges of fitting an item response theory model to the Social Anhedonia Scale. *Journal of Personality Assessment*, **93**(3), 213–24.

Richter, J., Holz, L., Hesse, K., Wildgruber, D., Klingberg, S. (2019). Measurement of negative and depressive symptoms: Discriminatory relevance of affect and expression. *European Psychiatry*, **55**, 23–8.

Ribot, T. (1896). *La Psychologie des Sentiments*. Paris: Felix Alcan, pp. 43–9.

Saeedi, H., Addington, J., Addington, D. (2007). The association of insight with psychotic symptoms, depression, and cognition in early psychosis: a 3-year follow-up. *Schizophrenia Research*, **89**(1–3), 123–8.

Schlier, B., Jaya, E. S., Moritz, S., Lincoln, T. M. (2015). Validation of the Community Assessment of Psychic Experiences (CAPE) in a community and clinical sample. *Schizophrenia Research*, **169**(1–3), 274–9.

Selten, J. P., Wiersma, D., Van Den Bosch, R. J. (2000). Clinical predictors of discrepancy between self-ratings and examiner ratings for negative symptoms. *Comprehensive Psychiatry*, **41**(3), 191–6.

Selten, J. P., Sijben, N. E., Van Den Bosch, R. J., Omloo-Visser, J., Warmerdam, H. (1993). The subjective experience of negative symptoms: a self-rating scale. *Comprehensive Psychiatry*, **34**(3), 192–7.

Sevy, S., Nathanson, K., Visweswaraiah, H., Amador, X. (2004). The relationship between insight and symptoms in schizophrenia. *Comprehensive Psychiatry*, **45**(1), 16–19.

Stefanis, N. C., Hanssen, M., Smirnis, N. K., Avramopoulos, D. A., Evdokimidis, I., Stefanis, C. N. (2002). Evidence that three dimensions of psychosis have a distribution in the general population. *Psychological Medicine*, **32**(2), 347–58.

Strauss, G. P., Nunez, A., Ahmed, A. O., Barchard, K. A., Granholm, E., Kirkpatrick, B., et al. (2018). The latent structure of negative symptoms in schizophrenia. *JAMA Psychiatry*, **75**(12), 1271–9.

Thaker, G., Moran, M., Adami, H., Cassady, S. (1993). Psychosis proneness scales in schizophrenia spectrum personality disorders: familial vs. nonfamilial samples. *Psychiatry Research*, **46**(1), 47–57.

Tso, I. F., Grove, T. B., Taylor, S. F. (2014). Differential hedonic experience and behavioral activation in schizophrenia and bipolar disorder. *Psychiatry Research*, **219**(3), 470–6.

Upthegrove, R., Birchwood, M., Ross, K., Brunett, K., McCollum, R., Jones, L. (2010). The evolution of depression and suicidality in first episode psychosis. *Acta Psychiatrica Scandinavica*, **122**(3), 211–18.

Wild, D., Grove, A., Martin, M., Eremenco, S., McElroy, S., Verjee-Lorenz, A., et al. (2005). Principles of good practice for the translation and cultural adaptation process for patient-reported outcomes (PRO) measures: report of the ISPOR Task Force for Translation and Cultural Adaptation. *Value Health*, **8**(2), 94–104.

CHAPTER 4

CHAPTER 5

Pharmacologic treatment of negative symptoms: Focus on efficacy

Pál Czobor and István Bitter

KEY POINTS

- During the last decade, negative symptoms in schizophrenia have been recognized by regulatory agencies as a legitimate indication for potential drug targets.
- Significant progress has been made to improve measurement of negative symptoms and to distinguish between primary and secondary negative symptoms by controlling for 'pseudospecific' effects in clinical trials.
- To deal with the problem of pseudospecificity, regulators and academic experts underline the importance of focusing on patients with predominant negative symptoms in pharmacological studies of negative symptoms.
- Nonetheless, there have been only very few clinical trials that focused on patients with predominant negative symptoms.
- A large meta-analysis found that second-generation antipsychotics (SGA) had the greatest efficacy for negative symptoms, followed by first-generation antipsychotics (FGA), combination treatments, antidepressants, and glutamatergic medications. The included studies, however, were not specifically designed to measure negative symptoms.
- With respect to patients with predominant negative symptoms, in the largest trial conducted so far, the recently approved SGA antipsychotic, cariprazine was superior to its SGA antipsychotic comparator, risperidone.
- For medication classes other than antipsychotics and antidepressants, we found no reliable support that would substantiate evidence-based recommendations for using these agents in the treatment of negative symptoms in clinical practice.

5.1 Introduction

Treatment of negative symptoms constitutes a major challenge and unmet need for schizophrenia. Evidence indicates that negative symptoms are associated with worse quality of life and poorer functional outcomes than positive symptoms (Sarkar, Hillner, and Velligan, 2015). Thus, selecting the best available treatment to target negative symptoms could lead to important improvements in the psychosocial functioning of patients suffering from schizophrenia. Accumulating data show that currently available psychopharmacological treatments with FGA and SGA antipsychotics have major limitations in terms of reducing negative symptoms (Sarkar, et al. 2015). Thus, pharmacologists, drug developers, and treating clinicians are in a renewed search to identify efficient psychopharmacological approaches that show promise for clinically important benefits in the treatment of negative symptoms. In this chapter, we will first briefly review some of the critical issues and milestone changes that took place during the last ten years in the regulatory and clinical environment. These changes are important as they fundamentally determined the course of drug development and the type of data that are being collected in clinical trials to support the efficacy claims for negative symptom treatments.

We will then present an overview of a comprehensive meta-analytic comparison of various classes of drugs (antipsychotics, antidepressants, glutamatergic agent, and combination of antipsychotic and combination treatments) with respect to their efficacy in the treatment of negative symptoms. Following this, we will provide a summary of the empirical data for antipsychotics in the treatment of negative symptoms. Finally, we review the clinical trial evidence for some of the most important classes of therapeutic agents that are considered to be potentially beneficial for negative symptoms. We classified the therapeutic agents according to psychiatric medication class (antipsychotics, antidepressants, CNS stimulants, anticonvulsants) or on the basis of their site of action or mechanism of action (glutamatergic, cholinesterase inhibitors, anti-inflammatory and immuno-modulatory agents, sex hormones). Our goal was to concentrate on the highest level of evidence. Therefore, we relied on meta-analyses and review articles available for a given area since they summarize data from multiple studies; data from single studies are shown only when they provide critical supplementary information.

5.2 Recent milestones in the clinical trial environment for the assessment therapeutic benefits for negative symptoms

In this section, we review four milestone changes that occurred in the last ten years in the area of regulatory environment and negative symptom research that fundamentally determined the clinical trial settings for negative symptom studies.

The first milestone was the endorsement from the US Food and Drug Administration (FDA) that negative symptoms can be considered as legitimate targets for drug development for schizophrenia. Agency representatives stated that while the FDA generally discourages drug developments that focus narrowly on certain features of a defined psychiatric syndrome when other drugs are considered to be treatments for the broad syndrome, it nonetheless makes exceptions when there is a legitimate basis for targeting selected aspects of a psychiatric disorder (Laughren and Levin, 2011). To meet this requirement, psychiatrists need to provide empirical evidence that negative symptoms of schizophrenia represent a specific feature of the illness. In the absence of such evidence, the FDA would consider the claim regarding negative symptoms as 'pseudospecific', that is, not sufficiently distinct from other aspects of the illness (e.g. cognitive and depressive symptoms, extrapyramidal side effects) (Laughren and Levin, 2011).

The second milestone pertains to the measurement of negative symptoms, and was coming from experts in the negative symptoms field. Specifically, based on a consensus of experts, it has been stipulated that the original negative symptom items on the Positive and Negative Syndrome Scale (PANSS; Kay, Fiszbein, and Opler, 1987) or the Brief Psychiatric Rating Scale (BPRS; Overall and Gorham, 1962) anergia factor do not provide adequate representation of negative symptoms; instead, the PANSS negative factors that emerged from factor analyses are preferred. In addition, there was also a consensus that studies should report a global rating of negative symptoms in addition to the scale scores. Furthermore, if a scale does not include a global measure of negative symptoms then an external global measure of negative symptoms should be added as an additional item (Marder, Daniel, Alphs, et al. 2011). Currently, besides the PANSS negative symptom factors, the NSA-16 (Axelrod, Goldman, and Alphs, 1993), the CAINS (Clinical Assessment Interview for Negative Symptoms, by NIMH Collaboration to Advance Negative Symptom Assessment in Schizophrenia, CANSAS) (Kring et al. 2013), and the BNSS (Brief Negative Symptom Scale) are used in clinical studies (Kirkpatrick, Strauss, Nguyen, et al. 2011).

The third milestone is the requirement that treatments for negative symptoms need to exhibit efficacy against 'primary' negative symptoms because improvement on 'secondary' negative symptoms may be 'pseudo-specific', that is, the consequence of improvements on other symptom dimension (e.g. depressive symptoms). In order to address this problem, the European Medicines Agency (EMA) explicitly stated that patients with predominant negative symptoms should be included in such studies (European Medicines Agency and Committee for Medicinal Products for Human Use (CHMP), 2012). These patients, as described elsewhere in this book in more detail, are required to have a substantial burden from negative symptoms with the additional criteria of no-to-little severity of positive symptoms. Nonetheless, there is still a debate whether clinical trial populations should also include patients with prominent negative symptoms (Marder, Alphs, Anghelescu, et al. 2013). Patients with prominent negative symptoms are characterized as patients with a high degree of negative symptoms, who also may exhibit a substantial burden from positive symptoms. Unfortunately, as we will see in this chapter, so far there have been very few clinical studies that focused on primary negative symptoms and selected chronically ill patients with predominant or prominent negative symptoms. Furthermore, the evidence is primarily coming from short-term studies, which do not allow judgement about the efficacy with regard to the persistency of the therapeutic effects.

The fourth milestone was the specification of clinical trial designs by the regulatory agency that may provide evidence for beneficial therapeutic effects in negative symptom studies. Two trial designs were considered by the US regulatory agency (Laughren and Levin, 2006).

The first trial design is a 'Switch trial, for a broad-spectrum agent (BSA)'. This would include a run-in period during which patients would be stabilized on a standard antipsychotic agent (SA), and then in a double blind phase they would continue with randomization to either staying on that SA or switching to the new BSA. The anticipated outcome would be an improvement in negative symptoms on the BSA and no change in negative symptoms in patients continuing on the SA. However, the interpretation of the results would not be straightforward (e.g. both the BSA and the SA cause negative symptoms; however, the BSA has a lesser effect on inducing negative symptoms, so that patients appear to improve when switched to the BSA).

The second trial design is an 'Add-on trial'. This would be used for an agent to specifically target negative symptoms in patients whose positive symptom are controlled with an antipsychotic drug and who would continue on that drug during the negative symptom trial to maintain control of the positive symptoms. For the Add-on trial, two approaches could be implemented. The first approach is to use a single identified drug (i.e. the new drug is added on to a single identified standard drug). According to FDA policy, the single standard drug design would require that the FDA's combination policy be met; that is, it would be necessary to show that the combination of new investigational drug and a standard drug is superior to each drug alone. The second approach is to use an all-comers approach (patients stabilized on one of several standard antipsychotics are randomized). The FDA would require a two-arm trial of new drug or placebo added on to the standard, because the alternative design of testing all combinations against all single-dose arms would not be feasible.

5.3 Comprehensive meta-analysis of psychopharmacological treatments of negative symptom treatments: findings of a meta-analysis of 168 randomized placebo-controlled trials

The meta-analysis we describe here (Fusar-Poli, Papanastasiou, Stahl, et al. 2015) examined whether there are any effective treatments for negative symptoms and compared various interventions (pharmacological as well as psychological) with respect to their efficacy. Here, we focus on the relevant results with respect to pharmacological treatments, which included FGAs and SGAs, glutamatergic medications, antidepressants (AD), and combinations of these medications. The analysis included all randomized placebo-controlled trials for negative symptoms in schizophrenia published up to December 2013. The primary efficacy measures included the Negative Symptom Subscale of the Positive and Negative Syndrome Scale (PANSS) for Schizophrenia (Kay, et al. 1987), the Withdrawal-Retardation Subscale of the Brief Psychiatric Rating Scale (Overall and Gorham, 1962), and the Scale for the Assessment of Negative Symptoms (SANS; Andreasen, 1982). Treatment efficacy was expressed in terms of Cohen-D effect size versus placebo. Specifically, this effect size measure expresses the mean difference in the primary outcome measures (i.e. the mean difference between the post- and pre-treatment score) between treatment and placebo groups in a standardized form, by dividing the mean treatment group difference by the pooled standard deviation (SD) of the difference scores.

The analysis dataset comprised data from a total of 6,503 patient in the treatment arms and from 5,815 patients in the placebo arms of the included studies. Pharmacological treatments produced improvements in negative symptoms which were either statistically significant (in case of SGA, AD, glutamatergic medications (GLU), or combinations of psychopharmacological treatments), or a marginally significant (in case of FGAs). The largest effect size was associated with treatments with SGA medications (Cohen-D = −0.579). FGAs yielded the second largest effect size, even though the Cohen-D value was only marginally significant due to the smaller number of studies that included FGA antipsychotics. Combination treatments also elicited a robust reduction of negative symptoms with a Cohen-D effect size of −0.518. Antidepressants were associated with a small-to-medium effect size with a Cohen-D of −0.349, while glutamatergic medications yielded a statistically significant, but small effect (Cohen-D: −0.228).

The authors of the meta-analysis (Fusar-Poli, et al. 2015) considered the effects, mentioned earlier, on negative symptoms as clinically not meaningful. However, it is important to note that this meta-analysis yielded greater effect sizes for FGAs and SGAs and combination treatments for negative symptoms than placebo-controlled regulatory trials for acute schizophrenia yielded for total symptom severity (which includes positive and negative symptoms and general psychopathology). Furthermore, the effect size for negative symptoms was greater than the effect size that is achieved in most clinical trials of antidepressant medications.

Additionally, there are several issues that require consideration with respect to these data. First, some of the measures that were used in the individual studies (e.g. BPRS Anergia factor) were not endorsed by experts in the field (as they are not sufficiently specific to measure negative symptoms). Second, based on the available data primary and secondary negative symptoms could not be separated. Third, most of the studies were conducted before 2013, that is before expert recommendations for the currently recognized target population for trials of patients with negative symptoms have been stipulated (e.g. inclusion of patients with predominant or prominent negative symptoms).

Fourth, some of the Cohen-D values for the meta-analysis were computed using the standard errors (instead of the standard deviations) (Leucht et al. 2017), which could have confounded the findings.

5.4 Antipsychotic medications in the treatment of negative symptoms

We identified three meta-analyses which provided detailed data on improvements of negative symptoms in clinical studies of antipsychotics. The first two analyses were based on trials that were not designed to specifically investigate negative symptoms: one compared FGAs and SGAs (Leucht, Corves, Arbter, et al. 2009a), while the other one compared several SGAs with each other (Leucht, Komossa, Rummel-Kluge, et al. 2009b). The third meta-analysis was based on trials which focused on predominant or prominent negative symptoms (Krause Zhu, Huhn, et al. 2018).

Effects of FGAs versus SGAs on negative symptoms. This meta-analysis (Leucht, et al. 2009a) compared oral formulations of nine SGAs (amisulpride, aripiprazole, clozapine, olanzapine, quetiapine, risperidone, sertindole, ziprasidone, and zotepine) with first-generation drugs on various measures of efficacy, including improvement on negative symptoms. The analyses were based on data from 21,533 patients diagnosed with schizophrenia or related disorders (including schizoaffective, schizophreniform, or delusional disorders). These patients were enrolled in a total of 150 mostly short-term, double blind studies, published up to October 2006. The study concluded that four SGAs (amisulpride, clozapine, olanzapine, and risperidone) had significantly greater efficacy than the FGAs had with respect to negative symptoms. These drugs were also more efficacious than FGAs for the treatment of positive symptoms.

Comparison of effects of various SGAs on negative symptoms. This meta-analysis (Leucht, et al. 2009b) was a pairwise comparison of various SGAs used in the treatment of schizophrenia. The meta-analysis was based on data from a total of 13,558 participants from 78 studies, published up to September 2007. The primary outcome measure was the change in total score on the Positive and Negative Syndrome Scale; the negative symptom subscale score was a secondary measure. The SGAs that were included in this meta-analysis were amisulpride, aripiprazole, clozapine, olanzapine, quetiapine, risperidone, sertindole, ziprasidone, and zotepine. This meta-analysis revealed differences among SGAs in terms of overall efficacy. Specifically, olanzapine had greater efficacy than aripiprazole, quetiapine, risperidone, and ziprasidone. Risperidone was superior to quetiapine and ziprasidone, and clozapine was superior to zotepine and, in doses > 400 mg/day, to risperidone. However, these differences were associated with changes in positive symptoms. With the exception of two small studies, there were no significant differences with regard to negative symptoms.

Summary of the findings from the two earlier meta-analyses. Taken together, the first two meta-analyses, conducted by Leucht and co-workers (Leucht, Corves, Arbter, et al. 2009a; Leucht, Komossa, Rummel-Kluge, et al. 2009b) highlight that SGAs achieve significantly better efficacy than FGAs in the treatment of negative symptoms, but there are no significant differences among SGAs (with the exception of cariprazine which we will discuss later). However, based on the lack of specificity of outcome measures in these short-term studies that included patients with acute exacerbations of positive symptoms of schizophrenia, it remains unclear whether these studies reflect that antipsychotics improve only the 'secondary' or also the 'primary' negative symptoms. It is conceivable that the reduction of negative symptoms was attributable to the amelioration of positive or depressive symptoms or to the reduction of extrapyramidal side effects of prior treatments which could mimic negative symptoms.

Antipsychotic drugs for patients with predominant or prominent negative symptoms. The meta-analysis described here (Krause, et al. 2018) focused on antipsychotic medications. This analysis is particularly important since its selection criteria were based on the aforementioned regulatory agency and expert panel recommendations and used data from patients with either predominant or prominent negative symptoms. In the included studies, negative symptoms were investigated as the primary outcome. They were measured by the negative subscale of the PANSS (PANSS-negative), the SANS, or by other validated scales for the assessment of negative symptoms in schizophrenic patients (e.g. BNSS). To account for the potential impact of secondary negative symptoms, depressive and positive symptoms, and extrapyramidal side effects were also analysed.

The meta-analysis included all available data (published up until the end of 2017) for all 34 FGAs or SGAs which were licensed in the United States or at least one country in Europe, and were seen as important by a survey of international schizophrenia experts. In the included studies these antipsychotics were used as monotherapy (at any dose and in any form of administration), and were compared with another antipsychotic or placebo. The authors conducted separate pairwise analyses between individual antipsychotics.

Using the pairwise comparison approach, there were 9 out of 21 studies that included patients with predominant negative symptoms and yielded data for the selected negative symptom measures. The investigated treatments included amisulpride, sulpiride, asenapine, cariprazine, clozapine, flupentixol, fluphenazine, haloperidol, olanzapine, placebo, quetiapine, risperidone, ziprasidone, and zotepine. We note that only four of the nine treatments were tested in more than one study; these were amisulpride ($n = 4$), olanzapine ($n = 3$), quetiapine ($n = 3$), and risperidone ($n = 3$). Patients with prominent negative symptoms were examined in 12 of the 21 studies. These studies focused on the following drugs: amisulpride, clozapine, flupentixol, fluphenazine, haloperidol, olanzapine, quetiapine, risperidone, sulpiride, ziprasidone and zotepine. Once again, only 4 of 12 treatments were tested in more than two studies: amisulpride ($n = 4$), olanzapine ($n = 3$), quetiapine ($n = 3$), and risperidone ($n = 3$). Thus, the number of studies available for the analysis of both the prominent and the predominant negative symptom trials was small.

With regard to prominent negative symptoms, there was only one placebo-controlled study among the included studies. This indicated a difference between sulpride and placebo (less improvement for sulpride), which reached the level of statistical significance ($p = 0.05$). Direct comparisons between antipsychotics showed significant treatment differences in negative symptom improvements in two trials. In one of these studies, in terms of standardized mean difference (SMD) olanzapine was superior to risperidone ($n = 235$, SMD $= -0.30$); and in a rather small trial quetiapine outperformed risperidone (total $n = 44$, SMD $= -1.34$). No significant difference was found in pairwise comparisons between olanzapine and quetiapine; clozapine and haloperidol; and risperidone and flupenthixol. In these studies, several significant treatment-related changes emerged in various symptom dimensions in addition to the improvements on negative symptoms. Thus, studies of patients with prominent negative symptoms could have been confounded by changes in other symptom dimensions. This problem was alleviated in studies of patients with predominant negative symptoms where these potential confounders were exclusion criteria, and a minimum threshold severity for the relevant negative symptoms was required.

With respect to predominant negative symptoms, only three drugs (amisulpride, olanzapine, zotepine) were compared with placebo. Based on the respective pairwise comparisons, amisulpride was significantly better than placebo based on four trials ($n = 590$, SMD $= 0.47$). Based on a single trial, olanzapine was not significantly more efficacious than placebo and its effect size was close to zero with respect to negative symptoms. Zotepine did not statistically significantly outperform placebo in a small trial (total $n = 35$), even though its effect size versus placebo was in the range of that of amisulpride (SMD $= 0.48$).

Direct comparisons of antipsychotics in patients with predominant negative symptoms indicated no significant difference between amisulpride and olanzapine and between asenapine and olanzapine in the improvement on negative symptoms. With respect to other comparisons between active treatments, the results indicated that olanzapine was significantly superior to haloperidol for negative symptoms in a small trial ($n = 35$, SMD $= 0.75$) while the SMDs did not show statistically significant difference for depression and positive symptoms.

In the largest trial performed so far for patients with predominant negative symptoms (total $n = 456$), the recently approved SGA antipsychotic cariprazine was significantly superior to its SGA antipsychotic comparator, risperidone (Nemeth, Laszlovszky, Czobor, et al. 2017). Cariprazine is a dopamine D3 and D2 receptor partial agonist, with a preference for the D3 receptor which is considered to be important in modulating mood and cognition, and may be beneficial in treating negative symptoms, dysphoria, and cognitive impairment in schizophrenia. Cariprazine is also a partial agonist at the serotonin 5-HT1A receptor and it acts as an antagonist at 5-HT2B and 5-HT2A receptors (Citrome, 2016). Cariprazine's effect size of superiority against risperidone in terms of SMD was -0.29, while no difference was observed between these drugs in terms of depressive and positive symptoms. This therapeutic effect therefore is noteworthy in terms of its specificity, since it was observed in the absence of the potential confounding effect of the relevant covariates, and was obtained in a large population. However, as pointed out by the authors of the meta-analysis, this study was conducted by the sponsor.

5.5 Antidepressants

Treatment of schizophrenia patients with negative symptoms often relies on the use of various add-on medications, including antidepressants. The synergistic effects of antipsychotics and antidepressants, especially selective serotonin re-uptake inhibitors (SSRIs), may be due to an increased dopamine release after administration of SSRI-antipsychotics, although other mechanisms of action including changes in γ-aminobutyric acid A (GABAA) receptor and related signal-ling systems have also been proposed in the literature (Potvin, Stip, Sepehry, et al. 2008, Silver, Susser, Danovich, et al. 2011). Based on empirical evidence, add-on trials with antidepressants for the treatment of depressive and negative symp-toms are approved by several treatment guidelines (e.g. APA guidelines, (Lehman, Lieberman, Dixon, et al.2004)).

As mentioned earlier, a meta-analysis (Fusar-Poli, et al. 2015) of randomized placebo-controlled trials of negative symptoms in schizophrenia indicates that antidepressants are associated with a small-to-medium effect size with a Cohen-D of -0.349. A recent meta-analysis (Helfer, Samara, Huhn, et al. 2016) focused specifically on add-on trials of antidepressants added to antipsychotics. The meta-analysis was based on a total of 3,608 participants' data, collected in 82 ran-domized controlled trials. Add-on antidepressants elicited statistically significant improvements in various symptom domains (negative, depressive, positive, total). The largest effect size was observed for negative symptoms, with a standardized mean difference of -0.30. The effect size for depressive and positive symptoms in terms of SMD was -0.25 and -0.17, respectively. Adjunctive antidepressant and control treatments did not differ with respect to the exacerbation of psych-osis during the study and in the proportion of patients who had at least one adverse event.

The effect size for adjunctive antidepressants increased when the minimum initial severity inclusion threshold for the target symptoms (negative and depres-sive symptoms) was increased. In particular, for studies which included patients with predominant negative symptoms the effect size was -0.58 as compared with -0.23 for the rest of the studies. Overall, the meta-analytic data suggest that the combination of antidepressants and antipsychotics can be effective in treating the negative symptoms of schizophrenia. The observed small, beneficial effects occur without an increase in the likelihood of exacerbation of psychotic symptoms, and at a low risk of adverse effects.

5.6 CNS stimulants

The modified dopamine (DA) hypothesis of schizophrenia posits that increased DA activity in the mesolimbic tract is associated with positive symptoms whereas decreased DA activity in the mesocortical prefrontal cortex may underlie nega-tive and cognitive symptoms (Howes and Kapur, 2009). Stimulant medications, such as amphetamine-based agents that are used in treatment of attention deficit hyperactivity disorder (ADHD) may increase the neuronal release of dopamine or norepinephrine, or (as in the case of modafinil or armodafinil) increase dopa-mine levels in the prefrontal cortex while reducing dopaminergic activity in the striatum (Lindenmayer, Nasrallah, Pucci, et al. 2013; Andrade, Kisely, Monteiro, et al. 2015). Thus, in view of the proposed role of DA in the pathogenesis of negative symptoms, stimulants that either directly or indirectly increase prefrontal dopaminergic neurotransmission have been hypothesized to improve negative symptoms. Based on this assumption, these agents have been investigated in clinical studies, despite the fact that historically they have been considered contraindicated due to their potential role in the exacerbation of positive symptoms.

Several reports have been published so far about the beneficial effects of various stimulant medications (e.g. d-amphetamine, methylphenidate) in the treatment of negative symptoms (Remington, Foussias, Fervaha, et al. 2016; Aleman, Lincoln, Bruggeman, et al. 2017). However, meta-analytic summary from controlled studies is available only for modafinil/armodafinil (Andrade, et al. 2015). This was based on data from 322 patients who were included in 6 randomized, controlled trials. The results indicated a statistically significant, but modest effect for modafinil/armodafinil in the improvement of negative symptoms (SMD = −0.26). The modafinil/armodafinil group did not differ from the placebo group in terms of dropout rates, and other outcome variables such as cognition, fatigue, daytime drowsiness, and adverse events. Thus, stimulant medications may have a potential role in the treatment of negative symptoms after a careful consideration of the potential risks and benefits of these drugs for individuals with schizophrenia.

5.7 Glutamate system

Dysregulation of the central nervous system glutamatergic activity is considered to contribute to the pathophysiology of schizophrenia (Kinon, Millen, Zhang, et al. 2015). Alterations in the glutamate system may be due to a hypofunction of the glutamate N-methyl-D-aspartate acid (NMDA) receptor (Veerman, Schulte, Smith, et al. 2016; Arango, Garibaldi, Marder, et al. 2013). Such an NMDA receptor hypofunction can be secondary to reduced inhibitory influences of the GABA system; this would result in a hyperstimulation of glutamatergic pyramidal neurons, possibly leading to neurotoxic effects.

NMDA-receptor coagonists. The possibility that NMDA-receptor coagonists may compensate for the hypofunction of the NMDA receptor led to an interest in investigational drugs that would work through this mechanism. Two meta-analyses (Tuominen Tiihonen, and Wahlbeck, 2005; Singh and Singh, 2011) which focused on drugs that enhance NMDA receptor function (e.g., D-serine, sarcosine, N-acetyl-cysteine, D-cycloserine) suggested that these drugs may elicit beneficial effects on negative symptoms. However, it should be noted that the effects were not consistent across the various agents (Singh and Singh, 2011).

NMDA receptor antagonists. Evidence that GABA may be increased, instead of being reduced, in unmedicated schizophrenia patients (Kegeles, Mao, Stanford, et al. 2012), and subjects at ultra-high risk (Fuente-Sandoval, Reyes-Madrigal, Mao, et al. 2015) led to trials of NMDA receptor antagonists in patients with schizophrenia (Aleman, et al. 2017). Overviewing the respective evidence, two meta-analyses focused on amantadine and memantine (Matsuda, Kishi, and Iwata,

2013; Kishi, Matsuda, and Iwata, 2017). Amantadine is an FDA approved drug with multiple indications (including Parkinson's disease), which is a weak antagonist at the NMDA-type glutamate receptor, blocks dopamine reuptake, and increases dopamine release. Memantine has uncompetitive NMDA receptor open-channel blocker properties and is indicated for Alzheimer's disease. It has been considered as a potentially promising add-on therapy for enhancing the clinical effectiveness of an on-going treatment with antipsychotics (Aleman, et al. 2017), especially clozapine (Veerman, Schulte, Begemann, et al. 2014). Nonetheless, with respect to negative symptoms, the two above-mentioned meta-analyses (Matsuda, Kishi, and Iwata, 2013; Kishi, Matsuda, and Iwata, 2017) did not provide a consistent support for the efficacy of these drugs. However, it should be noted that a more recent study reported a large effect size in an add-on trial of memantine for negative symptoms in schizophrenia (Rezaei, Mohammad-Karimi, Seddighi, et al. 2013).

Glycine. In addition to the NMDA receptor agonist or antagonist mechanism, the activity the NMDA system can be modulated through glycine receptors. Adopting this approach, endogenous glycine, N-acetyl-cysteine (NAC), and the agents D-serine and D-cycloserine have been studied as add-on medications to antipsychotics (Aleman, et al. 2017). A meta-analysis (Singh and Singh, 2011) showed that NAC, D-serine, and sarcosine as adjuncts to nonclozapine antipsychotics can be beneficial in the treatment of negative and total symptoms of chronic schizophrenia. However, a recent overview of placebo controlled schizophrenia trials of D-cycloserine showed inconsistent findings. For both clozapine and nonclozapine antipsychotics, improvement, or no change or even worsening of negative symptoms occurred in the various individual studies after add-on D-cycloserine treatment (Goff, 2017). With regard to glycine addition to clozapine, no effects on negative symptoms were identified by another meta-analysis (Evins, Fitzgerald, Wine, et al. 2000). However, it is important to note that there may be an optimal level of activity through the NMDA receptor, explaining the contradictory effects of addition strategies to clozapine, in comparison to other antipsychotics (Veerman, et al. 2014).

Specifically, clozapine may also act on the glutamate system and therefore add-on strategies additionally targeting the glutamate system through the NMDA receptor may exceed the optimal levels of glutamatergic stimulation. Nevertheless, the findings for glutamatergic agents are contradictory (Aleman, et al. 2017). For example, a large clinical trial of D-cycloserine and glycine revealed no significant effect for these agents (Buchanan, Javitt, Marder, et al. 2007). In fact, with respect to D-cycloserine, it has been raised that it may even increase negative symptoms through competition with endogenous glycine. Furthermore, the treatment strategy to increase the glycine levels through a selective glycine re-uptake inhibition by bitopertin failed in phase III after promising signals in earlier stages of the development (Bugarski-Kirola, et al. 2014).

Anticonvulsants with modulating effects on the glutamate and GABAergic systems. Several anticonvulsants which have a complex cellular mechanism of action may also modulate the glutamate and GABAergic systems (Aleman, et al. 2017). These drugs, including lamotrigine, valproate, topiramate, and carbamazepine, are being used as mood stabilizers in psychiatric practice, and have been investigated as potential add-on treatments to enhance the effects of antipsychotics in schizophrenia. For lamotrigine as an add-on treatment to clozapine, one meta-analysis showed some evidence for improving negative symptoms (Tiihonen, Wahlbeck, and Kiviniemi, 2009). However, a subsequent meta-analysis based on six studies of lamotrigine and four studies of topimarate did not indicate a significant effect on negative symptoms (Veerman, et al. 2014). In addition, as concluded by a review based on a small number of studies, the addition of topiramate, valproate, or carbamazepine to antipsychotics other than clozapine did not produce an effect on negative symptoms (Jiawan, Arends, Slooff, et al. 2010).

5.8 Cholinesterase inhibitors

Cholinesterase inhibitors represent a relatively new class of compounds which are being investigated for the treatment of schizophrenia. Cholinesterase inhibitors inhibit the cholinesterase enzyme system from breaking down acetylcholine, thereby increasing the level and duration of action of the neurotransmitter acetylcholine. Acetylcholine plays an important role in cognition, and impaired cholinergic transmission contributes to the cognitive deficits in Alzheimer's disease (Winkler, Thal, Gage, et al. 1998). A meta-analysis of adjunctive pharmacotherapy for cognitive deficits in schizophrenia showed a beneficial effect on certain cognitive functions and negative symptoms with two cholinesterase inhibitor drugs that are indicated in the treatment of Alzheimer's disease: donepezil and galantamine (the latter also acts as positive allosteric modulator of nicotine acetylcholine receptors) (Choi, Wykes, and Kurtz, 2013).

A review which specifically focused on cholinesterase inhibitors in schizophrenia also suggested that these drugs added to an antipsychotic show significant benefits over the antipsychotic plus placebo in negative symptom outcomes (Singh, Kour, and Jayaram, 2012). However, it should be noted that negative symptoms were not the primary outcome in the studies included in the meta-analysis, and no randomized controlled trials have been conducted with cholinesterase inhibitors so far that focused specifically on negative symptoms (Remington, et al. 2016). Furthermore, the interactions of the effects of changes in the negative symptoms and other symptom domains were not addressed in these meta-analyses. Finally, recent pharmacological development focused on newer $\alpha 7$ nicotinic acetylcholine receptor ($\alpha 7$ nAChR) agonists/partial agonists and positive allosteric modulators (Pohanka, 2012; Beinat, Banister, Herrera, et al. 2015), but at this point the clinical benefits of this research are difficult to evaluate in light of the negative results and the discontinuation of several early phase agents that act through the $\alpha 7$ nAChR system (Remington, et al. 2016).

5.9 Anti-inflammatory—immuno-modulatory agents

Potential utility of anti-inflammatory and immuno-modulatory treatments for schizophrenia is based on several lines of evidence (Muller, Weidinger, Leitner, et al. 2015; Rodrigues-Amorim, Rivera-Baltanas, Spuch, et al. 2017; Melbourne, Feiner, Rosen, et al. 2017). These include the observation of increased levels of pro-inflammatory substances such as cytokines that can be found in the blood and cerebrospinal fluid of schizophrenia patients. Moreover, blood cytokine abnormalities have been associated with poor cognitive function, regional brain volume alterations, and negative symptoms. The vulnerability—stress—inflammation model of schizophrenia (Zubin and Spring, 1977) considers the contribution of stress on the basis of increased genetic vulnerability for schizophrenia. Stress may lead to an elevation of pro-inflammatory cytokines and contribute to a chronic pro-inflammatory state. Such immune alterations influence the dopaminergic, serotonergic, noradrenergic, and glutamatergic neurotransmitter systems. In addition, it is important to note that antipsychotic drugs have intrinsic anti-inflammatory and immune-modulatory effects. Finally, added support for the inflammatory hypothesis comes from the therapeutic benefit of anti-inflammatory medications. For example, meta-analytic evidence exists about the beneficial effects of cyclo-oxygenase-2 (COX-2) inhibitors in early stages of schizophrenia (Muller, et al. 2015).

Drugs, other than COX-2 inhibitors, that have potential neuroprotective effects also hold out the promise for the treatment of negative symptoms. Among these compounds, minocycline needs to be mentioned because it has been submitted to testing in clinical trials that were specifically designed to investigate negative symptoms (Remington, et al. 2016; Aleman, et al. 2017). Minocycline is a broad-spectrum tetracycline antibiotic with neuroprotective properties, which are mediated through anti-inflammatory, anti-apoptotic, and antioxidant effects (Plane, Shen, Pleasure, et al. 2010). Minocycline may also modulate the NMDA or AMPA (α-amino-3-hydroxy-5-methyl-4-isoxazolepropionic acid) receptors and may protect against glutamate neurotoxicity. Several randomized double-blind placebo-controlled clinical trials reported improvement on add-on minocycline in terms of negative symptoms in patients with schizophrenia (Liu, Guo, Wu, et al. 2014; Kelly, Sullivan, McEvoy, et al. 2015). Although the sample size in these randomized trials was small (330 patients in 4 studies), a meta-analysis (Oya, Kishi, and Iwata, 2014) provided support for minocycline's beneficial effects for the treatment of negative symptoms in schizophrenia.

Among several other classes of drugs that lead to immune response modulation (e.g. nonsteroidal anti-inflammatory drugs (NSAIDs), acetylsalicylic acid (ASA)), statins received considerable attention in recent clinical trials as potential new treatments for schizophrenia. Statins, which are typically used as lipid-lowering drugs, are also proposed for promoting neuroprotection as a result of immune response modulation, blood flow regulation, oxidative damage reduction (van der Most, Dolga, Nijholt, et al. 2009), and anti-inflammatory effects

(Chen, Hung, Chen, et al. 2007; Gouveia Scorza, Silva, et al. 2011). While the results are inconsistent for statins as a broader class, a recently published study with the change on the PANSS negative symptom subscale score as the single primary measure of efficacy indicated significantly greater improvement for the add-on simvastatin than for the antipsychotic comparator, risperidone group (Tajik-Esmaeeli, Moazen-Zadeh, Abbasi, et al. 2017). These results were observed in the absence of significant changes in the PANSS positive symptom and general psychopathology subscale scores, and the severity of Hamilton Depression Scale and Extrapyramidal Symptom Rating Scale scores.

5.10 Sex hormones

Gender differences are manifested in schizophrenia in terms of virtually all major characteristics of schizophrenia including incidence and prevalence, age of onset, course of illness, symptom manifestation, and response to treatment. Hormones associated with sex differentiation during prenatal development have major effects on neuronal development, and there is evidence that these hormones influence sex differences in brain abnormalities in patients with schizophrenia. For example, it has been hypothesized that oestrogen can provide a protective role during female development, safeguarding against damage to brain regions that may have a critical role in schizophrenia (prefrontal cortex, amygdala, and hippocampus) (Rich and Caldwell, 2015; Buchanan, Kelly, Weiner, et al. 2017). Oestrogen enhances the secretion of oxytocin and the expression of its receptor, the oxytocin receptor, in the brain. Oxytocin is a 9-amino acid peptide hormone, synthesized primarily in neurons of the hypothalamic supraoptic and paraventricular nuclei, which promote social behaviour. In women, a single dose of estradiol has been found to be sufficient to increase circulating oxytocin concentrations (Acevedo-Rodriguez, Mani, and Handa, 2015).

Relationships between negative symptoms and various sex hormones have been reported in several studies (Remington, et al. 2016; Aleman, et al. 2017). For example, in randomized controlled trials positive results were reported for dehydroepiandrosterone (DHEA) (an adrenal hormone involved in the production of androgens and oestrogens); for the neurosteroid pregnenolone; and raloxifene, an oestrogen receptor modulator (Ritsner, Bawakny, and Kreinin, 2014). The latter agent reduced negative symptoms in post-menopausal females with schizophrenia who had prominent negative symptoms (Usall, Huerta-Ramos, Labad, et al. 2016). Recently, based on findings that oxytocin can promote social behaviour (Teng, Nonneman, Agster, et al. 2013) intranasal administration of oxytocin has been investigated in several trials as a potential add-on treatment for reducing negative symptoms. Results of these trials are promising even though some inconsistency remains. In particular, six of seven trials in patients with schizophrenia reported before 2016 found a reduction of negative symptoms after the use of oxytocin, although the possible long-term effects require further investigation (Feifel, Shilling, and MacDonald, 2016). However, a trial that was published more recently failed to observe a significant effect of oxytocin on negative symptoms (Dagani, Sisti, Abelli, et al. 2016), and in an updated meta-analysis oxytocin did not obtain statistical significance for reducing negative symptoms as compared to placebo, although the effect size for negative symptoms in each trial was associated with oxytocin dose.

5.11 Conclusion

During the last decade, landmark changes occurred in the regulatory, academic and clinical research environments in order to facilitate the search for efficient treatments for negative symptoms. Regulatory agencies recognized negative symptoms as legitimate indication for potential drug targets and specified possible trial designs for the demonstration of their efficacy. Major progress has also been made to better define and measure negative symptoms; and to distinguish between primary and secondary negative symptoms by controlling for 'pseudospecific' effects that occur due to changes in other symptom domains. To deal with the issue of pseudospecificity, regulators and academic experts underlined the importance of focusing on patients with predominant and enduring negative symptoms. Nonetheless, this progress has not yet been sufficiently represented in recent clinical trials. There are only very few clinical studies that focused on patients with predominant negative symptoms.

A large meta-analysis based on short-term trials of FGA and SGA, glutamatergic medications, antidepressants, and combinations of these medications found that SGA showed the greatest efficacy versus placebo, followed by FGA and combination treatments (all of these treatments demonstrated a medium effect size, with a Cohen-D between 0.5 and 0.58). Antidepressants yielded a small-to-medium effect (Cohen-D = -0.349), while glutamatergic medications produced small effect (Cohen-D: -0.228). However, the included studies were not specifically designed for negative symptoms, and did not specifically focus on patients with predominant negative symptoms. A recently published meta-analysis examined treatment effects of antipsychotic drugs based on data from patients with predominant or prominent negative symptoms. Unfortunately, the number of studies and number of patients included in the meta-analysis was small.

Direct comparisons between antipsychotics in patients with prominent negative symptoms showed significant treatment differences in negative symptom improvements in two trials. In one of these, olanzapine was superior to risperidone, and in a small trial quetiapine outperformed risperidone. Direct comparisons of antipsychotics in patients with predominant negative symptoms indicated that olanzapine was significantly superior to haloperidol for negative symptoms. In the largest trial conducted so far for patients with predominant negative symptoms (total $n = 456$), the recently approved SGA antipsychotic cariprazine was significantly superior to its SGA antipsychotic comparator, risperidone. However, as it has been pointed out, this study was conducted by the sponsor.

In this chapter we reviewed the clinical trial evidence for some of the potentially relevant classes of therapeutic agents (other than antipsychotics) that have been considered beneficial for the treatment of negative symptoms. These included antidepressants, CNS stimulants, anticonvulsants, glutamatergic agents, cholinesterase inhibitors, anti-inflammatory and immuno-modulatory agents, and sex hormones. Antidepressants showed a small to medium effect size among the classes; this result was replicated by a second meta-analysis. Based on currently available data, we found no reliable support for any of the other classes that would substantiate evidence based recommendations for using these agents in clinical practice. Future research should therefore continue the search for potential therapeutic interventions for primary negative symptoms, which remains an unmet clinical need.

REFERENCES

Acevedo-Rodriguez, A., Mani, S. K., Handa, R. J. (2015). Oxytocin and estrogen receptor beta in the brain: an overview. *Front Endocrinol (Lausanne)* **6**, 160.

Aleman, A., Lincoln, T. M., Bruggeman, R., Melle, I., Arends, J., Arango, C., et al. (2017). Treatment of negative symptoms: Where do we stand, and where do we go? *Schizophrenia Research*, **186**, 55–62.

Andrade, C., Kisely, S., Monteiro, I., Rao, S. (2015). Antipsychotic augmentation with modafinil or armodafinil for negative symptoms of schizophrenia: systematic review and meta-analysis of randomized controlled trials. *Journal of Psychiatric Research*, **60**, 14–21.

Andreasen, N. C. (1982). Negative symptoms in schizophrenia. Definition and reliability. *Archives in General Psychiatry*, **39**, 784–8.

Arango, C., Garibaldi, G., Marder, S. R. (2013). Pharmacological approaches to treating negative symptoms: a review of clinical trials. *Schizophrenia Research*, **150**, 346–52.

Axelrod, B. N., Goldman, R. S., Alphs, L. D. (1993). Validation of the 16-item Negative Symptom Assessment. *Journal of Psychiatric Research*, **27**, 253–8.

Beinat, C., Banister, S. D., Herrera, M., Law, V., Kassiou, M. (2015). The therapeutic potential of alpha7 nicotinic acetylcholine receptor (alpha7 nAChR) agonists for the treatment of the cognitive deficits associated with schizophrenia. *CNS Drugs*, **29**, 529–42.

Buchanan, R. W., Javitt, D. C., Marder, S. R., Schooler, N. R., Gold, J. M., McMahon, R. P., et al. (2007). The Cognitive and Negative Symptoms in Schizophrenia Trial (CONSIST): the efficacy of glutamatergic agents for negative symptoms and cognitive impairments. *American Journal of Psychiatry*, **164**, 1593–602.

Buchanan, R. W., Kelly, D. L., Weiner, E., Gold, J. M., Strauss, G. P., Koola, M. M., et al. (2017). A randomized clinical trial of oxytocin or galantamine for the treatment of negative symptoms and cognitive impairments in people with schizophrenia. *Journal of Clinical Psychopharmacology*, **37**, 394–400.

Bugarski-Kirola, D., Wang, A., Abi-Saab, D., Blattler, T. (2014). A phase II/III trial of bitopertin monotherapy compared with placebo in patients with an acute exacerbation of schizophrenia—results from the CandleLyte study. *European Neuropsychopharmacology*, **24**, 1024–36.

Chen, S. F., Hung, T. H., Chen, C. C., Lin, K. H., Huang, Y. N., Tsai, H. C., et al. (2007). Lovastatin improves histological and functional outcomes and reduces inflammation after experimental traumatic brain injury. *Life Sciences*, **81**, 288–98.

Choi, K. H., Wykes, T., Kurtz, M. M. (2013). Adjunctive pharmacotherapy for cognitive deficits in schizophrenia: meta-analytical investigation of efficacy. *British Journal of Psychiatry*, **203**, 172–8.

Citrome, L. (2016). Cariprazine for the treatment of schizophrenia: a review of this dopamine D3-preferring D3/D2 receptor partial agonist. *Clinical Schizophrenia and Related Psychoses*, **10**, 109–19.

Dagani, J., Sisti, D., Abelli, M., Di, P. L., Pini, S., Raimondi, S., et al. (2016). Do we need oxytocin to treat schizophrenia? A randomized clinical trial. *Schizophrenia Research*, **172**, 158–64.

European Medicines Agency, Committee for Medicinal Products for Human Use (CHMP) (2012). Guideline on clinical investigation of medicinal products, including depot preparations in the treatment of schizophrenia: Committee for Medicinal Products for Human Use (CHMP).

Evins, A. E., Fitzgerald, S. M., Wine, L., Rosselli, R., Goff, D. C. (2000). Placebo-controlled trial of glycine added to clozapine in schizophrenia. *American Journal of Psychiatry*, **157**, 826–8.

Feifel, D., Shilling, P. D., MacDonald, K. (2016). A Review of Oxytocin's Effects on the Positive, Negative, and Cognitive Domains of Schizophrenia. *Biological Psychiatry*, **79**, 222–33.

Fuente-Sandoval, C., Reyes-Madrigal, F., Mao, X., Leon-Ortiz, P., Rodriguez-Mayoral, O., Solis-Vivanco, R., et al. (2015). Cortico-striatal GABAergic and glutamatergic dysregulations in subjects at ultra-high risk for psychosis investigated with proton magnetic resonance spectroscopy. *International Journal of Neuropsychopharmacology*, **19**, yv105.

Fusar-Poli, P., Papanastasiou, E., Stahl, D., Rocchetti, M., Carpenter, W., Shergill, S., et al. (2015). Treatments of negative symptoms in schizophrenia: meta-analysis of 168 randomized placebo-controlled Trials. *Schizophrenia Bulletin*, **41**, 892–9.

Goff, D. C. (2017). D-cycloserine in schizophrenia: new strategies for improving clinical outcomes by enhancing plasticity. *Current Neuropharmacology*, **15**, 21–34.

Gouveia, T. L., Scorza, F. A., Silva, M. J., Bandeira, T. A., Perosa, S. R., Arganaraz, G. A., et al. (2011). Lovastatin decreases the synthesis of inflammatory mediators in the hippocampus and blocks the hyperthermia of rats submitted to long-lasting status epilepticus. *Epilepsy & Behavior*, **20**, 1–5.

Helfer, B., Samara, M. T., Huhn, M., Klupp, E., Leucht, C., Zhu, Y., et al. (2016). Efficacy and safety of antidepressants added to antipsychotics for schizophrenia: a systematic review and meta-analysis. *American Journal of Psychiatry*, **173**, 876–86.

Howes, O. D., Kapur, S. (2009). The dopamine hypothesis of schizophrenia: version III-- the final common pathway. *Schizophrenia Bulletin*, **35**, 549–62.

Jiawan, V. C., Arends, J., Slooff, C. J., Knegtering, H. (2010). [Pharmacological treatment of negative symptoms in schizophrenia; research and practice]. *Tijdschrift voor psychiatrie*, **52**, 627–37.

Kay, S. R., Fiszbein, A., Opler, L. A. (1987). The positive and negative syndrome scale (PANSS) for schizophrenia. *Schizophrenia Bulletin*, **13**, 261–76.

Kegeles, L. S., Mao, X., Stanford, A. D., Girgis, R., Ojeil, N., Xu, X., et al. (2012). Elevated prefrontal cortex gamma-aminobutyric acid and glutamate-glutamine levels in schizophrenia measured in vivo with proton magnetic resonance spectroscopy. *Archives in General Psychiatry*, **69**, 449–59.

Kelly, D. L., Sullivan, K. M., McEvoy, J. P., McMahon, R. P., Wehring, H. J., Gold, J. M., et al. (2015). Adjunctive minocycline in clozapine-treated schizophrenia patients with persistent symptoms. *Journal of Clinical Psychopharmacology*, **35**, 374–81.

Kinon, B. J., Millen, B. A., Zhang, L., McKinzie, D. L. (2015). Exploratory analysis for a targeted patient population responsive to the metabotropic glutamate 2/3 receptor agonist pomaglumetad methionil in schizophrenia. *Biological Psychiatry*, **78**, 754–62.

Kirkpatrick, B., Strauss, G. P., Nguyen, L., Fischer, B. A., Daniel, D. G., Cienfuegos, A., et al. (2011). The brief negative symptom scale: psychometric properties. *Schizophrenia Bulletin*, **37**, 300–5.

Kishi, T., Matsuda, Y., Iwata, N. (2017). Memantine add-on to antipsychotic treatment for residual negative and cognitive symptoms of schizophrenia: a meta-analysis. *Psychopharmacology (Berlin)*, **234**, 2113–25.

Krause, M., Zhu, Y., Huhn, M., Schneider-Thoma, J., Bighelli, I., Nikolakopoulou, A., et al. (2018). Antipsychotic drugs for patients with schizophrenia and predominant or prominent negative symptoms: a systematic review and meta-analysis. *European Archives in Psychiatry and Clinical Neurosciences*, **268**, 625–39.

Kring, A. M., Gur, R. E., Blanchard, J. J., Horan, W. P., Reise, S. P. (2013). The Clinical Assessment Interview for Negative Symptoms (CAINS): final development and validation. *American Journal of Psychiatry*, **170**, 165–72.

Laughren, T., Levin, R. (2006). Food and Drug Administration perspective on negative symptoms in schizophrenia as a target for a drug treatment claim. *Schizophrenia Bulletin*, **32**, 220–2.

Laughren, T., Levin, R. (2011). Food and Drug Administration commentary on methodological issues in negative symptom trials. *Schizophrenia Bulletin*, **37**, 255–6.

Lehman, A. F., Lieberman, J. A., Dixon, L. B., McGlashan, T. H., Miller, A. L., Perkins, D. O., et al. (2004). Practice guideline for the treatment of patients with schizophrenia, second edition. *American Journal of Psychiatry*, **161**, 1–56.

Leucht, S., et al. (2017). *American Journal of Psychiatry*, **174**, 927–42. doi: 10.1176/appi.ajp.2017.16121358

Leucht, S., Corves, C., Arbter, D., Engel, R. R., Li, C., Davis, J. M. (2009a). Second-generation versus first-generation antipsychotic drugs for schizophrenia: a meta-analysis. *Lancet*, **373**, 31–41.

Leucht, S., Komossa, K., Rummel-Kluge, C., Corves, C., Hunger, H., Schmid, F., et al. (2009b). A meta-analysis of head-to-head comparisons of second-generation antipsychotics in the treatment of schizophrenia. *American Journal of Psychiatry*, **166**, 152–63.

Lindenmayer, J. P., Nasrallah, H., Pucci, M., James, S., Citrome, L. (2013). A systematic review of psychostimulant treatment of negative symptoms of schizophrenia: challenges and therapeutic opportunities. *Schizophrenia Research*, **147**, 241–52.

Liu, F., Guo, X., Wu, R., Ou, J., Zheng, Y., Zhang, B., et al. (2014). Minocycline supplementation for treatment of negative symptoms in early-phase schizophrenia: a double blind, randomized, controlled trial. *Schizophrenia Research*, **153**, 169–76.

Marder, S. R., Daniel, D. G., Alphs, L., Awad, A. G., Keefe, R. S. (2011). Methodological issues in negative symptom trials. *Schizophrenia Bulletin*, **37**, 250–4.

Marder, S. R., Alphs, L., Anghelescu, I. G., Arango, C., Barnes, T. R., Caers, I., et al. (2013). Issues and perspectives in designing clinical trials for negative symptoms in schizophrenia. *Schizophrenia Research*, **150**, 328–33.

Matsuda, Y., Kishi, T., Iwata, N. (2013). Efficacy and safety of NMDA receptor antagonists augmentation therapy for schizophrenia: an updated meta-analysis of randomized placebo-controlled trials. *Journal of Psychiatric Research*, **47**, 2018–20.

Melbourne, J. K., Feiner, B., Rosen, C., Sharma, R. P. (2017). Targeting the immune system with pharmacotherapy in schizophrenia. *Current Treatment Options in Psychiatry*, **4**, 139–51.

Muller, N., Weidinger, E., Leitner, B., Schwarz, M. J. (2015). The role of inflammation in schizophrenia. *Frontiers in Neurosciences*, **9**, 372.

Nemeth, G., Laszlovszky, I., Czobor, P., Szalai, E., Szatmari, B., Harsanyi, J., et al. (2017). Cariprazine versus risperidone monotherapy for treatment of predominant negative symptoms in patients with schizophrenia: a randomised, double-blind, controlled trial. *Lancet*, **389**, 1103–13.

Overall, J. E., Gorham, D. R. (1962). The brief psychiatric rating scale. *Psychological Reports*, **10**, 799–812.

Oya, K., Kishi, T., Iwata, N. (2014). Efficacy and tolerability of minocycline augmentation therapy in schizophrenia: a systematic review and meta-analysis of randomized controlled trials. *Human Psychopharmacology*, **29**, 483–91.

Plane, J. M., Shen, Y., Pleasure, D. E., Deng, W. (2010). Prospects for minocycline neuroprotection. *Archives of Neurology*, **67**, 1442–8.

Pohanka, M. (2012). Alpha7 nicotinic acetylcholine receptor is a target in pharmacology and toxicology. *International Journal of Molecular Sciences*, **13**, 2219–38.

Potvin, S., Stip, E., Sepehry, A. A., Gendron, A., Bah, R., Kouassi, E. (2008). Inflammatory cytokine alterations in schizophrenia: a systematic quantitative review. *Biological Psychiatry*, **63**, 801–8.

Remington, G., Foussias, G., Fervaha, G., Agid, O., Takeuchi, H., Lee, J., et al. (2016). Treating negative symptoms in schizophrenia: an update. *Current Treatment Options in Psychiatry*, **3**, 133–50.

Rezaei, F., Mohammad-Karimi, M., Seddighi, S., Modabbernia, A., Ashrafi, M., Salehi, B., et al. (2013). Memantine add-on to risperidone for treatment of negative symptoms in patients with stable schizophrenia: randomized, double-blind, placebo-controlled study. *Journal of Clinical Psychopharmacology*, **33**, 336–42.

Rich, M. E., Caldwell, H. K. (2015). A role for oxytocin in the etiology and treatment of schizophrenia. *Frontiers in Endocrinology (Lausanne)*, **6**, 90.

Ritsner, M. S., Bawakny, H., Kreinin, A. (2014). Pregnenolone treatment reduces severity of negative symptoms in recent-onset schizophrenia: an 8-week, double-blind, randomized add-on two-center trial. *Psychiatry and Clinical Neurosciences*, **68**, 432–40.

Rodrigues-Amorim, D., Rivera-Baltanas, T., Spuch, C., Caruncho, H. J., Gonzalez-Fernandez, A., Olivares, J. M., et al. (2017). Cytokines dysregulation in schizophrenia: a systematic review of psychoneuroimmune relationship. *Schizophrenia Research*, July, **197**, 19–33.

Sarkar, S., Hillner, K., Velligan, D. I. (2015). Conceptualization and treatment of negative symptoms in schizophrenia. *World Journal of Psychiatry*, **5**, 352–61.

Silver, H., Susser, E., Danovich, L., Bilker, W., Youdim, M., Goldin, V., et al. (2011). SSRI augmentation of antipsychotic alters expression of GABA(A) receptor and related genes in PMC of schizophrenia patients. *International Journal of Neuropsychopharmacology*, **14**, 573–84.

Singh, J., Kour, K., Jayaram, M. B. (2012). Acetylcholinesterase inhibitors for schizophrenia. *Cochrane Database of Systematic Reviews*, **1**, CD007967.

Singh, S. P., Singh, V. (2011). Meta-analysis of the efficacy of adjunctive NMDA receptor modulators in chronic schizophrenia. *CNS Drugs*, **25**, 859–85.

Tajik-Esmaeeli, S., Moazen-Zadeh, E., Abbasi, N., Shariat, S. V., Rezaei, F., Salehi, B., et al. (2017). Simvastatin adjunct therapy for negative symptoms of schizophrenia: a randomized double-blind placebo-controlled trial. *International Clinical Psychopharmacology*, **32**, 87–94.

Teng, B. L., Nonneman, R. J., Agster, K. L., Nikolova, V. D., Davis, T. T., Riddick, N. V., et al. (2013). Prosocial effects of oxytocin in two mouse models of autism spectrum disorders. *Neuropharmacology*, **72**, 187–96.

Tiihonen, J., Wahlbeck, K., Kiviniemi, V. (2009). The efficacy of lamotrigine in clozapine-resistant schizophrenia: a systematic review and meta-analysis. *Schizophrenia Research*, **109**, 10–14.

Tuominen, H. J., Tiihonen, J., Wahlbeck, K. (2005). Glutamatergic drugs for schizophrenia: a systematic review and meta-analysis. *Schizophrenia Research*, **72**, 225–34.

Usall, J., Huerta-Ramos, E., Labad, J., Cobo, J., Nunez, C., Creus, M., et al. (2016). Raloxifene as an adjunctive treatment for postmenopausal women with schizophrenia: a 24-week double-blind, randomized, parallel, placebo-controlled trial. *Schizophrenia Bulletin*, **42**, 309–17.

van der Most, P. J., Dolga, A. M., Nijholt, I. M., Luiten, P. G., Eisel, U. L. (2009). Statins: mechanisms of neuroprotection. *Progress in Neurobiology*, **88**, 64–75.

Veerman, S. R., Schulte, P. F., Begemann, M. J., Engelsbel, F., de Haan, L. (2014). Clozapine augmented with glutamate modulators in refractory schizophrenia: a review and metaanalysis. *Pharmacopsychiatry*, **47**, 185–94.

Veerman, S. R., Schulte, P. F., Smith, J. D., de Haan, L. (2016). Memantine augmentation in clozapine-refractory schizophrenia: a randomized, double-blind, placebo-controlled crossover study. *Psychological Medicine*, **46**, 1909–21.

Winkler, J., Thal, L. J., Gage, F. H., Fisher, L. J. (1998). Cholinergic strategies for Alzheimer's disease. *Journal of Molecular Medicine (Berlin)*, **76**, 555–67.

Zubin, J., Spring, B. (1977). Vulnerability--a new view of schizophrenia. *Journal of Abnormal Psychology*, **86**, 103–26.

CHAPTER 6

Psychosocial/non-pharmacologic treatment of negative symptoms: Focus on efficacy

Mark Savill

KEY POINTS

- In a series of meta-analyses social skills training, music therapy, non-invasive brain stimulation, mindfulness, and exercise-based interventions have all been found to improve negative symptoms in randomized controlled trials, relative to treatment as usual.
- Effect sizes for these interventions range from small to moderate.
- More work is necessary to evaluate the long-term benefits of these interventions.
- The evidence for arts therapies other than music therapy, CBTp, neurocognitive therapies, and family-based interventions is more inconsistent.
- Although statistically significant, there has been some debate as to whether these interventions lead to consistent, clinically meaningful change. As a result, primary negative symptoms of schizophrenia can still be considered an important unmet therapeutic need where more research is needed.

6.1 Introduction

Given the limited impact of current pharmacological treatments for negative symptoms (Leucht, Leucht, Huhn, et al. 2017), current best practice supports the use of psychological and psychological interventions in addition to medication (i.e. Kreyenbuhl, Buchanan, Dickerson, et al. 2010; NICE, 2010). In recognition of this, a number of non-pharmacological interventions have been proposed and evaluated. In the following chapter, we review the literature evaluating these interventions which include neurocognitive therapies, social skills training, cognitive behavioural therapy for psychosis (CBTp), non-invasive brain stimulation, exercise-based interventions, and arts therapies. A summary of the evidence will be based on a series of meta-analyses, which are presented in Table 6.1.

Table 6.1 Meta analytic studies examining the impact of treatments of negative symptoms of psychosis

Study	Number of Studies included	N	Effect size Estimates	95% CI	
Neurocognitive therapies					
Lutgens, et al. 2017	16	1208	−0.15	−0.41	0.11
Cella, et al. 2017	45	2511	−0.30*	−0.36	−0.22
Skills training					
Kurtz and Mueser, 2008	6	363	0.40*	0.19	0.61
Lutgens, et al. 2017	17	775	−0.44*	−0.77	−0.10
Cognitive Behaviour Therapy					
Wykes, et al. 2008	23	1268	0.44*	0.17	0.70
Jauhar, et al. 2014	34	2354	−0.13	0.25	−0.01
Velhorst, et al. 2015	30	2312	0.09	−0.03	0.21
Mindfulness-based therapies					
Khoury, et al. 2013	3	111	0.56*	0.15	0.96
Exercise therapy					
Firth, et al. 2015	4	140	−0.44*	−0.78	−0.09
Lutgens, et al. 2017	10	581	−0.36*	−0.71	−0.01
Brain stimulation					
Aleman, et al. 2018	24	961	0.35*	0.16	0.53
Arts therapies					
NICE, 2009	6	382	−0.59*	−0.83	−0.36
Lutgens, et al. 2017	7	893	−0.14	−0.78	0.50
Lutgens, et al. 2017[†]	5	418	−0.58*	−0.82	−0.33
Geretsegger, et al. 2017[†]	3	177	−0.55*	−0.87	−0.24
Family-based interventions					
Lutgens, et al. 2017	3	177	−0.19	−0.7	0.34

Key: CI: confidence interval; * Mean difference to control at end of treatment significant at $p < 0.05$; [†]Music therapy only.

6.2 Neurocognitive therapies

Cognitive deficits inherent to psychosis typically refer to a range of impairments, including deficits in attention, working memory, verbal learning and memory, visual learning and memory, reasoning and problem solving, and social cognition (Nuechterlein, Barch, Gold, et al. 2004). While cognitive symptoms represent a distinct symptom cluster from negative symptoms, they are considered at least partially related, associated with slower processing speed, poorer abstract reasoning, impaired shift setting, and the poorer generation and execution of cognitive strategies (Heydebrand, Weiser, Rabinowitz, et al. 2004). As a result, it has been proposed that adopting interventions designed to treat cognitive impairment in psychosis may also lead to improvements in negative symptoms. Proposed mechanisms include improving working memory (Strauss and Gold, 2012), reward sensitivity (Cella, Preti, Edwards, et al. 2017), self-esteem (Kidd, Kaur, Virdee, et al. 2014) which may influence amotivation and experiential deficits, and improvements in executive functioning (Farreny, Aguado, Ochoa, et al. 2013).

'Neurocognitive therapies' include cognitive remediation, cognitive training, cognitive rehabilitation, neurocognitive therapy, and cognitive enhancement. These interventions typically adopt one of two distinct approaches, known as the 'drill and strategy coaching' and 'drill and practice' methods (McGurk, Twamley, Sitzer, et al. 2007). In drill and practice, participants engage in a range of cognitive tasks that get progressively more difficult as the participant improves, the rationale being that this leads to more efficient neural response which generalizes to other areas of cognition (Fisher, Holland, Merzenich, et al. 2009). In the drill and coaching strategy, the completion of these cognitive tasks is combined with additional input, such as the therapy to help identify triggers of cognitive impairment, and/or the teaching learning strategies that can be generalized to daily life.

A number of neurocognitive interventions have been used with people with psychosis. One extensively validated intervention following the 'drill and practice method includes the BrainHQ training program by PositScience (http://www.brainhq.com), while an example of the drill and strategy coaching method includes CIRCuiTS (Reeder and Wykes, 2010). While both treatments have been validated as a treatment for negative symptoms, these interventions were not primarily developed with this as the primarily target, and no neurocognitive treatments developed specifically for this purpose were identified.

6.2.1 Evidence of effectiveness

In a review of the literature, two recent meta-analyses evaluating the effectiveness of neurocognitive therapies on negative symptoms were identified (Cella, et al. 2017; Lutgens, Gariepy, and Malla, 2017). In the Lutgens study, over 16 studies, 11 evaluated cognitive remediation, 2 cognitive training, 1 cognitive rehabilitation, 1 neurocognitive therapy, and 1 cognitive enhancement. Six studies compared effects to treatment as usual (TAU), while active control groups across the remaining studies included computer games, supportive therapy, leisure activities, CBT, dance and music therapy, and generic group activities. Of the 16 studies, neurocognitive therapies were found to be an effective treatment for negative symptoms in 5 trials, and no significant effect overall was detected (SMD −0.15, 95% CI −0.41 to 0.11).

In the study by Cella and colleagues (2017), 45 studies that evaluated cognitive remediation specifically were identified. Of these, 15 were compared to TAU, and 30 compared to active controls including occupational therapy/vocational support, psyched programs, behavioural rehabilitation programs, CBT, skills training, leisure activities, group therapy/activities, video watching, music and dance therapy, and computer games/IT skills training. Cognitive remediation was found significantly to reduce negative symptoms related to control at both end of treatment (SMD 0.30, 95% CI 0.36 to 0.22) and at follow-up (SMD 0.36, 95% CI 0.51 to 0.21). This significant difference was consistent in studies that compared cognitive remediation to treatment as usual, and to an active control. A longer treatment duration was associated with marginally stronger treatment effects. Of note, the many of the high-quality studies that reported the largest effect size improvements incorporated an extensive coaching component which supported participants to apply the skills in everyday life.

6.2.2 Summary

In the meta-analysis that generalized across all neurocognitive therapies no significant effect was detected (Lutgens, et al. 2017). However, in a second larger review which focused on cognitive remediation specifically small to moderate improvements in negative symptoms were detected, with improvements maintained at follow-up (Cella, et al. 2017). In the second review, it was suggested that studies that incorporated a coaching component to support the application of these learnt skills in daily life resulted in greater improvements. This finding is consistent with an earlier review which reported that neurocognitive therapies that adopt the drill and coaching strategy yielded greater improvements in negative symptoms and related constructs (McGurk, et al. 2007). Consequently, the evidence suggests that neurocognitive therapies, when combined with additional skills training and therapy input, may be considered an effective treatment for negative symptoms.

6.3 Social skills training

Social skills training approaches are interventions designed to address impairments in social skills that are a common deficit in individuals with psychosis (Mueser, Bellack, Douglas, et al. 1991). Impairments in social skills are associated with more severe negative symptoms (Lysaker, Bell, Zito, et al. 1995), and poorer psychosocial adjustment (Bellack, Morrison, Wixted, et al. 1990; Mueser and Bellack, 1998). Consequently, interventions to address these deficits may represent an important strategy to address negative symptoms in psychosis (Kurtz and Mueser, 2008).

Different social skills training programmes vary significantly in their content, but they typically share strategies based on social learning theory (Bandura, 1969). These include goal setting, role modelling and role-play activities, positive reinforcement, and homework assignments (Kurtz and Mueser, 2008). Validated manuals for social skills training in schizophrenia are available for therapists and counsellors, the most extensively used being authored by Bellack and colleagues (Bellack, Mueser, Gingerich, et al. 2013). More recently, this work has extended into the field of neurocognitive therapies with the aim of addressing social cognitive deficits. In these interventions, the focus is on practising skills related to social cognitive processes (Kurtz, Gagen, Rocha, et al. 2016). However, while there is evidence to suggest that this training may improve social cognition and facial affect recognition, these changes have not been found to extend to negative symptoms (Kurtz and Richardson, 2012).

6.3.1 Evidence of effectiveness

Here the findings of two systematic reviews will be summarized. The first focused exclusively on social skills training, which required the inclusion of core behavioural techniques such as role play/rehearsal and corrective feedback (Kurtz and Mueser, 2008). The second adopted much broader criteria, incorporating skills training programmes, occupational therapy, and cognitive adaptation training (Lutgens, et al. 2017).

In the Kurtz and Meuser study, 23 studies were identified (Kurtz and Mueser, 2008). Of these, six evaluated the impact of social skills training on negative symptoms. The training was found to result in significant improvements in negative symptoms relative to control (SMD 0.40, 95% CI 0.19 to 0.61). There was some evidence to suggest that younger participant age was associated with a greater improvement in symptoms. In the Lutgens study, 17 studies were identified (Lutgens, et al. 2017). Of these, 11 evaluated skills training, 3 occupational therapy, 2 cognitive adaptation training, and 1 vocational training. Overall, these treatments were found to lead to significant improvements in negative symptoms relative to controls (SMD –0.44, 95% CI –0.77 to –0.10), with effects maintained up to six months later. In subgroup analyses, the effect size improvements were found to be substantially larger when compared to treatment as usual, relative to an active control.

6.3.2 Summary

Current findings suggest that social skills training may be an effective treatment for negative symptoms of psychosis. Furthermore, there is evidence to suggest that these improvements are maintained over time. The findings reported in the reviewed meta-analyses are consistent with those reported in a recent narrative synthesis evaluating psychosocial treatments for negative symptoms (Elis, Caponigro, and Kring, 2013).

6.4 Cognitive Behavioural Therapy for Psychosis (CBTp)

Cognitive behavioural therapy (CBT) is rooted in the premise that cognitive factors contribute to the development and maintainence of mental disorders (Beck, 1970). Consequently, stratagies that successfully modify maladaptive cognitions can lead to positive changes in behaviours, symptoms, and distress. While CBT was originally developed to treat affective disorders, in recent years the model has been adapted to treat psychotic disorders. In these CBT for psychosis (CBTp) models, the principle aim is to challenge maladaptive cognitions related to psychotic phenomena which is considered to be the cause of distress and functional impairment (Morrison, 2001).

While early CBTp interventions were developed to treat positive symptoms such as hallucination and delusions (Chadwick, Birchwood, and Trower, 1996; Garety, Kuipers, Fowler, et al. 2001), interventions have since been developed specifically to treat negative symptoms. (i.e. Klingberg, Wölwer, Engel, et al. 2011; Staring, ter Huurne, and van der Gaag, 2013). Both adopt general principles of CBT, including case formulation, goal setting, homework assignments, and role play. However, treatments designed to treat negative sympoms include a greater focus on self-stigma, discrimination and exclusion, mourning, and demoralization, with the aim of addressing defeatest beliefs (Klingberg, et al. 2011; Staring, ter Huurne, and van der Gaag, 2013). These interventions have been evaluated in both an individual and group format.

6.4.1 Evidence of effectiveness

CBTp is an accepted treatment for psychosis that has been recommended by the National Collaborating Centre for Mental Health (NCCMH)) for over 15 years (NCCMH, 2003). With regards to negative symptoms specifically, in a review completed by Wykes and colleagues (Wykes, Steel, Everitt, et al. 2008) 23 studies evaluating the impact of CBTp on negative symptoms were identified, which were found significantly to reduce negative symptoms relative to control (SMD 0.44, 95% CI 0.17 to 0.70). However, when only high-quality studies were considered, this difference was not found to be significant (SMD 0.21, 95% CI − 0.10 to 0.52). In two more recent reviews (Jauhar, McKenna, Radua, et al. 2014; Velthorst, Koeter, Van Der Gaag, et al. 2015), the significant effect on negative symptoms was either not present, or not found when only high-quality studies were included. The significantly lower effect sizes found in these studies were primarily attributed to the fact that more recent, higher-quality studies could not replicate the findings of earlier trials.

Looking to the future, it is unclear whether CBTp that focuses specifically on negative symptoms, as opposed to psychosis more broadly, may represent a more effective treatment strategy. This was examined in the review by Velthorst and colleagues (Velthorst, et al. 2015), but with insufficient studies evaluating reporting negative symptoms as a primary outcome no firm conclusions could be drawn. Two recent studies evaluating CBT interventions with a specific focus on dysfunctional expectancies about one's own abilities show promising results (Grant, Huh, Perivoliotis, et al. 2012; Staring, et al. 2013), suggesting this may be an important area for future exploration.

In terms of how the treatment should be delivered (i.e. individually or in groups), the results appeared inconsistent. In the Wykes review no difference was found in outcomes between the two modalities, however in the Velthorst review individual treatment was found to be significantly more effective than group therapy (SMD 0.21, in comparison to SMD −0.17, $p = 0.02$). Finally, in the Velthorst review there was some evidence to suggest that treatments that focused more heavily on behavioural techniques appeared to report larger effect sizes.

6.4.2 Summary

Recent meta-analytic studies suggest that CBTp for psychosis may not be as effective at reducing negative symptoms as once thought. At present, it is unclear if treatments adapted specifically to treat negative symptoms of psychosis represent a more effective treatment strategy. There is some evidence to suggest that CBTp delivered individually, as opposed to in a group format, and with a strong emphasis on behavioural techniques, may be more effective.

6.5 Mindfulness-based interventions

Mindfulness is a process rooted in Eastern (particularly Buddhist) traditions, and is defined as the self-regulation of attention on present experiences in an open, accepting, and curious manner (Bishop, Lau, Shapiro, et al. 2004). Different mindfulness interventions are typically based on meditative practice, acceptance based, or kindness and compassion based (Khoury, Lecomte, Fortin, et al. 2013). Consistent across these different interventions is the aim to regulate negative emotions through the acceptance, rather than avoidance or confrontation, of present experiences. In psychosis, this extends to experiencing positive symptoms in the moment as separate from the self, and transient in nature (Chadwick, Taylor, and Abba, 2005). With regards to negative symptoms specifically, mindfulness-based intervention such as loving-kindness meditation build on the broaden-and-build theory (Fredrickson, 2001), where the mindful thoughts towards positive relationships over time are thought to build personal resources (Johnson, Penn, Fredrickson, et al. 2009).

A number of different mindfulness-based treatment protocols have either been designed or adapted for use with individuals with psychosis. These include Loving Kindness Meditation (Salzberg, 1995; Brantley and Hanauer, 2008); Acceptance and Commitment therapy (Hayes, Strosahl, and Wilson, 1999), and Mindfulness-based Cognitive Therapy (Segal, Teasdale, and Williams, 2004).

6.5.1 Evidence of effectiveness

In a recent meta-analysis, three randomized controlled trials (RCTs) evaluating the impact of mindfulness on negative symptoms of psychosis were identified (Khoury, Lecomte, Fortin, et al. 2013). The control arms were either treatment as usual, or befriending. The review found that mindfulness significantly reduced negative symptoms as compared to control (SMD 0.56, 95% CI 0.15 to 0.96). However, the total sample size across the three studies was small ($n = 111$), indicating more evidence, particularly from full-scale trials, is needed. No follow-up data concerning negative symptoms specifically were reported, and so the long-term impacts of these interventions are also unclear.

6.5.2 Summary

In recent years mindfulness has gained significant traction as an intervention that can reduce symptoms and alleviate distress across a range of mental health disorders. At present, there is an insufficient evidence base evaluating mindfulness-based approaches as a treatment for negative symptoms of psychosis. However, a minimal but emerging evidence base of small-scale pilot studies do indicate promise. Looking to the future, full-scale RCTs evaluating the impact of mindfulness on negative symptoms of psychosis with an adequate period of follow-up may represent one important future direction for treatment and research. Given the focus on addressing negative symptoms and building personal resources, and kindness and compassion-based mindfulness approaches may represent the most promising avenue for the treatment of these symptoms, in the absence of more substantial evidence.

6.6 Non-invasive brain stimulation

Two methods of non-invasive brain stimulation designed to treat the negative symptoms include repetitive transcranial magnetic stimulation (rTMS) and transcranial direct current stimulation (tDCS). These interventions are thought to have two different mechanisms of action. In rTMS, neuronal firing is induced by supra-threshold neuronal membrane depolarization, while in tDCS neuronal activity is modulated via membrane polarization (Paulus, 2011; Aleman, Enriquez-Geppert, Knegtering, et al. 2018). In both cases, the treatment of negative symptoms via neurostimulation typically focuses in the dorsolateral prefrontal cortex (DLPFC). This area is thought to be critical in neurological models of goal-directed behaviour (Yamagata, Nakayama, Tanji, et al. 2012), and patients with negative symptoms typically experience decreased activation in this region (Wolkin, Sanfilipo, Wolf, et al. 1992). Where low-frequency rTMS is recommended as a treatment for positive symptoms (Wassermann and Lisanby, 2001), in negative symptoms high-frequency stimulation is supported to induce dopamine release and increase cortical excitation (Stanford, Corcoran, Bulow, et al. 2011).

Side effects of non-invasive brain stimulation are typically mild (headaches, mild pain at the stimulation site), although in very rare cases seizures have been reported. Consequently, brain stimulation should not be considered appropriate for individuals with a personal or familial history of seizures/epilepsy, or organic brain disorders (O'Reardon, Peshek, Romero, et al. 2006).

6.6.1 Evidence of effectiveness

In a recent systematic review evaluating the effectiveness of both rTMS and tDS as a treatment for negative symptoms 24 trials were identified (Aleman, Enriquez-Geppert, Knegtering, et al. 2018). Across both intervention types, non-invasive brain stimulation significantly reduced negative symptoms as compared to an active sham control, which was maintained even after removing outliers that found a particularly strong effect (SMD 0.35, 95% CI 0.16 to 0.53). When examined in isolation, both rTMS and tDS were found to lead to significant improvements relative to control. In an analysis of the potential moderators of the effect, younger age, shorter duration of illness, and greater number of sessions were found to be associated with larger effect sizes.

6.6.2 Summary

The current evidence suggests non-invasive brain stimulation represents an effective treatment for negative symptoms of psychosis, with moderate effect size improvements relative to sham control conditions detected. In future work, it is necessary to evaluate the effectiveness of these treatments over a longer follow-up period to determine whether these improvements can be maintained over the longer-term.

6.7 Arts therapies

The four main types of art therapy include fine art therapy, music therapy, dance movement/body psychotherapy, and drama therapy. In many countries, arts therapies are delivered by trained and certified therapists. Arts therapies typically adopt a process-oriented approach with a focus on the creative process, non-verbal communication, and on developing a safe space for expression (Payne, 1993). It has been argued that two features to art therapies in particular are advantageous to treating negative symptoms of psychosis. First, negative symptoms include deficits in the ability to express oneself verbally (Kirkpatrick, Fenton, Carpenter, et al. 2006), so the focus on non-verbal communication may represent an alternative avenue for expression less impacted by their disorder. Second, using creative methods may represent a safer method to explore and connect with powerful feelings and events that might otherwise overwhelm the patient (Crawford and Patterson, 2007).

6.7.1 Evidence of effectiveness

In 2009, NICE recommended arts therapies as a treatment for negative symptoms, based on promising findings in a series of small-scale trials (NICE, 2009). These recommendations were based on a systematic review conducted in 2007, were across six small-scale studies, and moderate-to-large effect sizes were found in favour of arts therapies relative to control both at end of treatment (SMD –0.59, 95% CI –0.83 to –0.36), and up to six months later. However, since the publication of this review two major RCTs, one in fine arts (Crawford, Killaspy, Barnes, et al. 2012) and one in body psychotherapy (Priebe, Savill, Wykes, et al. 2016) reported non-significant findings, leading to the effectiveness of these interventions being questioned.

More recently, attention has focused specifically on the impact of music therapy on negative symptoms. In two recent meta-analyses (Geretsegger, Mössler, Bieleninik, et al. 2017; Lutgens, et al. 2017) music therapy was found to be an effective treatment, while a third review found evidence of a dose response effect with more music therapy sessions leading to a greater reduction on negative symptoms (Gold, Solli, Krüger, et al. 2009). These findings suggest that music therapy may represent an effective treatment for negative symptoms. However, while these results are promising, more evidence from larger full-scale trials is necessary.

6.7.2 Summary

Following promising evidence from a series of small-scale trials, more recent full-scale clinical trials in body psychotherapy and fine arts therapy suggest that arts therapies as a singular entity may not represent an effective treatment for negative symptoms. However, there is some limited evidence to suggest that music therapy specifically may lead to significant improvements over treatment as usual, although more evidence is needed.

6.8 Family-based interventions

Family-based interventions for negative symptoms of psychosis typically consist of psychotherapy, psychoeducation, and skills training, delivered either in a multi-family group, single family, or a mixture of the two formats. These interventions focus on providing psychoeducation around psychosis and the treatment process, help families to understand and change existing dynamics within the family system, and assist families in developing peer support networks (Wynne, 1988; Dyck, Short, Hendryx, et al. 2000). In doing so, the aim is to modify family dynamics that may create or maintain problematic behaviours, and help families and patients improve coping and illness management skills.

Of the family-based interventions for psychosis, the most commonly adopted method is that originally developed by McFarlane and colleagues (McFarlane, Lukens, Dushay, et al. 1995). In an adaptation of the McFarlane model, Dyck and colleagues developed and evaluated a family-based intervention specifically designed to treat negative symptoms, delivered in a community setting (Dyck, et al. 2000).

6.8.1 Findings

While a number of studies evaluating the impact of family-based interventions were identified, many were delivered in conjunction with other psychosocial treatments. As a result, disentangling the impact of family interventions specifically based on the evidence is challenging. In a review by Lutgens and colleagues that evaluated family therapy delivered in isolation (Lutgens, et al. 2017), no significant improvement in negative symptoms was detected relative to a control (SMD −0.19, 95% CI −0.70 to 0.34). However, the review only included three relatively small studies (total $n = 168$), and so lacked power to identify any possible effect reliably. In a narrative synthesis which included studies where family therapy was delivered in combination with other treatment modalities (personal therapy, assertive community treatment, and/or skills training), the impact of treatment appeared more promising (Elis, et al. 2014). Of the nine studies identified in this review, six reported significant negative symptom improvements in the family intervention arms, relative to the control conditions, with differences maintained up to two years later. With regards to how the intervention should be delivered, there is some limited evidence to suggest that family interventions when delivered in a group, as opposed to a single setting may lead to significantly greater improvements in negative symptoms (McFarlane, et al. 1995)

6.8.2 Summary

At present, there is insufficient evidence to determine if family-based approaches represent an effective treatment for the negative symptoms of psychosis. Few evaluations of family-based approaches as a treatment for negative symptoms have been conducted, and when they have, they have often been evaluated in conjunction with other non-pharmacological treatments. Going forwards, more trials either evaluating the effectiveness of family-based interventions in isolation, or as an additive component, would be informative in determining the specific effects of this particular intervention. Additionally, clinical trials further evaluating the impact of family-based interventions delivered in a group format, as opposed to with individual families would be highly informative. While inconclusive, there is some evidence to suggest greater treatment effects when delivered in a group format (McFarlane, et al. 1995).

6.9 Exercise

In addition to traditional psychotherapeutic interventions, there is an emerging evidence base to suggest that exercise therapy may also represent an effective intervention to treat the negative symptoms of psychosis. Interventions that have been evaluated in this field include yoga (Duraiswamy, Thirthalli, Nagendra, et al. 2007; Varambally, Gangadhar, Thirthalli, et al. 2012), resistance training (Scheewe, Backx, Takken, et al. 2013), aerobic exercise (Acil, Dogan, and Dogan 2008), walking groups (Loh, Abdullah, Bakar, et al. 2016), tai chi (Ho, Au Yeung, Lo, et al. 2012), and team sports (i.e. football; Battaglia, Alesi, Inguglia, et al. 2013). Most are consistent with the World Health Organization (WHO) guidelines that measure activity guidelines around time spent exercising at moderate-to-vigorous level of activity (WHO, 2010). These interventions are typically delivered in a group setting by trained occupational or psychomotor specialists, although in some cases exercise has been prescribed in an unsupervised format (i.e. gym membership provision). When unsupervised, there is some preliminary evidence to suggest that dropout from activity may be higher (i.e. Acil, et al. 2008). Exercise represents a generic intervention, so, to date, no manuals have been specifically developed to treat negative symptoms.

In addition to treating negative symptoms, an added benefit to providing exercise therapy to patients with psychosis may alleviate some of the symptoms associated with the metabolic syndrome (De Hert, et al. 2009), which is associated with taking antipsychotics. Metabolic syndrome includes a cluster of symptoms including obesity, high blood pressure and hyperglycemia (Alberti, Zimmet, Shaw,. 2005). The impact of these symptoms are significant, with this decline in physical health linked to a reduce life expectancy in people with schizophrenia by 15–20 years (Laursen, 2011).

6.9.1 Evidence of effectiveness

In a literature research, two recent systematic reviews evaluating the impact of exercise therapy on negative symptoms of psychosis were identified (Firth, Cotter, Elliott, et al., 2015; Lutgens, et al. 2017). In the Firth review, across eight studies no significant effects of exercise were found on negative symptoms. However, in a subgroup analysis that included only studies which evaluated moderate-to-vigorous exercise ($k = 4$), significant negative symptom improvement across the intervention arms was detected (SMD = −0.44, 95% CI −0.78 to −0.09). In the Lutgens study, across all studies exercise interventions were found to lead to significant improvements in negative symptoms relative to control (SMD −0.36, 95% CI −0.71 to −0.01), with the effect more notable when compared to TAU as opposed to a physically active control which could potentially mask the effect of activity. In the Lutgens review, lower-quality studies reported a greater effect of exercise on negative symptoms, suggesting the need for larger, high-quality evaluations in the field. Since the publication of these reviews at least one more study has been published, in which high-intensity interval training was also found to significantly reduce negative symptoms in psychosis to waitlist control (Romain, Fankam, Karelis, et al. 2018).

6.9.10 Summary

A small, but emerging evidence base consistently supports the finding that exercise therapy may alleviate negative symptoms, with interventions leading to small-to-moderate effect size improvements relative to treatment as usual. However, at present the evidence base is relatively limited, and larger, high-quality studies are needed. In studies that evaluated unsupervised exercise high dropout rates were identified as a concern. In the future, it may be important to evaluate difference between group versus individual activity, and possible variations between the types of activity. In particular, further investigations into the effectiveness of moderate-to-vigorous activity, as opposed to light activity, may be merited. Based on current evidence, exercise interventions may represent a relatively low-cost intervention that may help reduce negative symptoms, and address some of the significant physical health complications that are associated with psychosis and long-term antipsychotic use.

6.10 Conclusion

Of the interventions reviewed, skills training, non-invasive brain stimulation, music therapy, and exercise therapy that incorporates at least moderate levels of activity were all found to improve negative symptoms significantly relative to a control, with small-to-medium effects sizes reported. More evidence is needed to determine the longer-term impact of these interventions, although there is evidence to suggest that the effects of skills training is maintained at least six months later.

Regarding other interventions, recent studies evaluating CBTp have failed to replicate the earlier promising findings, and so at present it is unclear whether this intervention represents a viable treatment strategy for negative symptoms. Further work may be necessary to evaluate CBTp approaches adapted to target negative symptoms specifically. With neurocognitive therapies, the 'drill and coaching strategy', where adjunctive coaching and support is provided, may be necessary for improvements to extend to negative symptoms. With family-based interventions, more evidence is needed before firm conclusions can be drawn, however multi-family group-based formats may result in greater improvements relative to single-family treatments. With body psychotherapy and fine art therapy, the initial promise of small-scale studies have not been replicated in full-scale trials, suggesting these approaches may not be an effective treatment for negative symptoms.

While a number of interventions have been found to lead to statistically significant improvements in negative symptoms, it is important to consider whether these represent clinically meaningful changes. In a recent meta-analysis, it has been suggested that the effect size improvements reported here do not constitute clinically meaningful changes in negative symptoms at a group level (Fusar-Poli, Papanastasiou, Stahl, et al. 2015). The relatively small effect size improvements suggest that primary negative symptoms of schizophrenia should still be considered an unmet therapeutic need, and an important target for new interventions (Kirkpatrick, et al. 2006).

In the future, there is some evidence to suggest that combining non-pharmacological interventions may lead to even greater effect size improvements, as has been identified in recent exploratory studies where cognitive training and aerobic exercise (Nuechterlein, Ventura, McEwen, et al. 2016) and CBT with social skills training (Granholm, Holden, and Worley, 2017) have been delivered concurrently. This is consistent with the approach increasingly adopted in the treatment of early psychosis, where comprehensive, multidisciplinary approaches that include multiple treatment elements have been found to improve clinical and functional outcomes significantly (Craig, Garety, Power, et al. 2004; Petersen, Nordentoft, Jeppesen, et al. 2005; Kane, Robinson, Schooler, et al. 2015).

REFERENCES

Acil, A. A., Dogan, S., Dogan, O. (2008). The effects of physical exercises to mental state and quality of life in patients with schizophrenia. *Journal of Psychiatric and Mental Health Nursing, 15*(10), 808–15.

Alberti, K. G. M., Zimmet, P., Shaw, J. (2005). The metabolic syndrome—a new worldwide definition. *The Lancet, 366*(9491), 1059–62.

Aleman, A., Enriquez-Geppert, S., Knegtering, H., Dlabac-de Lange, J. J. (2018). Moderate effects of noninvasive brain stimulation of the frontal cortex for improving negative symptoms in schizophrenia: meta-analysis of controlled trials. *Neuroscience & Biobehavioral Reviews, 89*, 111–18.

Bandura, A. (1969). *Principles of Behavior Modification.* New York: Holt, Rinehart and Winston.

Battaglia, G., Alesi, M., Inguglia, M., Roccella, M., Caramazza, G., Bellafiore, M., et. al. (2013). Soccer practice as an add-on treatment in the management of individuals with a diagnosis of schizophrenia. *Neuropsychiatric Disease and Treatment, 9*, 595–603.

Beck, A. T. (1970). Cognitive therapy: nature and relation to behavior therapy. *Behavior Therapy, 1*, 184–200.

Bellack, A. S., Mueser, K. T., Gingerich, S., Agresta, J. (2013). *Social Skills Training for Schizophrenia: A Step-by-Step Guide.* New York, Guilford Publications.

Bellack, A. S., Morrison, R. L., Wixted, J. T., Mueser, K. T. (1990). An analysis of social competence in schizophrenia. *British Journal of Psychiatry, 156*, 809–18

Bishop, S. R., Lau, M., Shapiro, S., Carlson, L., Anderson, N. D., Carmody, J., et al. (2004). Mindfulness: a proposed operational definition. *Clinical Psychology: Science and Practice, 11*(3), 230–41.

Brantley, M., Hanauer, T. (2008). *The Gift of Loving-Kindness: 100 Meditations on Compassion, Generosity, and Forgiveness.* Oakland, New Harbinger Publications.

Cella, M., Preti, A., Edwards, C., Dow, T., Wykes, T. (2017). Cognitive remediation for negative symptoms of schizophrenia: a network meta-analysis. *Clinical Psychology Review, 52*, 43–51.

Craig, T. K., Garety, P., Power, P., Rahaman, N., Colbert, S., Fornells-Ambrojo, M., Dunn, G. (2004). The Lambeth Early Onset (LEO) Team: randomised controlled trial of the effectiveness of specialised care for early psychosis. *British Medical Journal, 329*(7474), 1067.

Crawford, M. J., Patterson, S., 2007. Arts therapies for people with schizophrenia: an emerging evidence base. *Evidence-Based Mental Health, 10*(3), 69.

Chadwick, P. D., Birchwood, M. J., Trower, P. (1996). *Cognitive Therapy for Delusions, Voices and Paranoia.* Chichester, John Wiley & Sons.

Chadwick, P., Taylor, K. N., Abba, N. (2005). Mindfulness groups for people with psychosis. *Behavioural and Cognitive Psychotherapy, 33*(3), 351–9.

Crawford, M. J., Killaspy, H., Barnes, T. R., Barrett, B., Byford, S., Clayton, K., et al. (2012). Group art therapy as an adjunctive treatment for people with schizophrenia: multicentre pragmatic randomised trial. *British Medical Journal*, **344**, e846.

Duraiswamy, G., Thirthalli, J., Nagendra, H. R., Gangadhar, B. N. (2007). Yoga therapy as an add-on treatment in the management of patients with schizophrenia–a randomized controlled trial. *Acta Psychiatrica Scandinavica*, *116*(3), 226–32.

Dyck, D. G., Short, R. A., Hendryx, M. S., Norell, D., Myers, M., Patterson, T., et al. (2000). Management of negative symptoms among patients with schizophrenia attending multiple-family groups. *Psychiatric Services*, **51**(4), 513–19.

Elis, O., Caponigro, J. M., Kring, A. M. (2013). Psychosocial treatments for negative symptoms in schizophrenia: current practices and future directions. *Clinical Psychology Review*, *33*(8), 914–28.

Farreny, A., Aguado, J., Ochoa, S., Haro, J. M., Usall, J. (2013). The role of negative symptoms in the context of cognitive remediation for schizophrenia. *Schizophrenia Research*, *150*(1), 58–63.

Firth, J., Cotter, J., Elliott, R., French, P., Yung, A. R. (2015). A systematic review and meta-analysis of exercise interventions in schizophrenia patients. *Psychological Medicine* **45**(7), 1343–61.

Fisher, M., Holland, C., Merzenich, M. M., Vinogradov, S. (2009). Using neuroplasticity-based auditory training to improve verbal memory in schizophrenia. *American Journal of Psychiatry*, **166**, 805–11.

Fredrickson, B. L. (2001). The role of positive emotions in positive psychology. The broaden-and-build theory of positive emotions. *American Psychologist*, 56(3), 218–26.

Fusar-Poli, P., Papanastasiou, E., Stahl, D., Rocchetti, M., Carpenter, W., Shergill, S., et al. (2014). Treatments of negative symptoms in schizophrenia: meta-analysis of 168 randomized placebo-controlled trials. *Schizophrenia Bulletin*, *41*(4), 892–9.

Garety, P. A., Kuipers, E., Fowler, D., Freeman, D., Bebbington, P. E. (2001). A cognitive model of the positive symptoms of psychosis. *Psychological Medicine*, *31*(2), 189–95.

Geretsegger, M., Mössler, K. A., Bieleninik, Ł., Chen, X. J., Heldal, T. O., Gold, C. (2017). Music therapy for people with schizophrenia and schizophrenia-like disorders. *Cochrane Database of Systematic Reviews*, (5).

Gold, C., Solli, H. P., Krüger, V., Lie, S. A. (2009). Dose–response relationship in music therapy for people with serious mental disorders: Systematic review and meta-analysis. *Clinical Psychology Review*, **29**(3), 193–207.

Granholm, E., Holden, J., Worley, M. (2017). Improvement in negative symptoms and functioning in cognitive-behavioral social skills training for schizophrenia: mediation by defeatist performance attitudes and asocial beliefs. *Schizophrenia Bulletin*, **44**(3), 653–61.

Grant, P. M., Huh, G. A., Perivoliotis, D., Stolar, N. M., Beck, A. T. (2012). Randomized trial to evaluate the efficacy of cognitive therapy for low-functioning patients with schizophrenia. *Archives of General Psychiatry*, *69*(2), 121–7.

Hayes, S. C., Strosahl, K. D., Wilson, K. G. (1999). *Acceptance and Commitment Therapy* New York, Guilford Press.

De Hert, M., Schreurs, V., Vancampfort, D., Van Winkel, R. (2009). Metabolic syndrome in people with schizophrenia: a review. *World Psychiatry*, *8*(1), 15–22.

Heydebrand, G., Weiser, M., Rabinowitz, J., Hoff, A. L., DeLisi, L. E., Csernansky, J. G. (2004). Correlates of cognitive deficits in first episode schizophrenia. *Schizophrenia Research*, **68**(1), 1–9.

Ho, R. T., Au Yeung, F. S., Lo, P. H., Law, K. Y., Wong, K. O., Cheung, I. K., et. al. (2012). Tai-chi for residential patients with schizophrenia on movement coordination, negative symptoms, and functioning: a pilot randomized controlled trial. *Evidence-Based Complementary and Alternative Medicine*, 923925. pmid:23304224.

Jauhar, S., McKenna, P. J., Radua, J., Fung, E., Salvador, R., Laws, K. R. (2014). Cognitive–behavioural therapy for the symptoms of schizophrenia: systematic review and meta-analysis with examination of potential bias. *British Journal of Psychiatry* **204**(1), 20–9.

Johnson, D. P., Penn, D. L., Fredrickson, B. L., Meyer, P. S., Kring, A. M., Brantley, M. (2009). Loving-kindness meditation to enhance recovery from negative symptoms of schizophrenia. *Journal of Clinical Psychology*, *65*(5), 499–509.

Kane, J. M., Robinson, D. G., Schooler, N. R., Mueser, K. T., Penn, D. L., Rosenheck, R. A., et al. (2015). Comprehensive versus usual community care for first-episode psychosis: 2-year outcomes from the NIMH RAISE early treatment program. *American Journal of Psychiatry*, *173*(4), 362–72.

Khoury, B., Lecomte, T., Fortin, G., Masse, M., Therien, P., Bouchard, V., et al. (2013). Mindfulness-based therapy: a comprehensive meta-analysis. *Clinical Psychology Review*, *33*(6), 763–71.

Kidd, S. A., Kaur, J., Virdee, G., George, T. P., McKenzie, K., Herman, Y. (2014). Cognitive remediation for individuals with psychosis in a supported education setting: A randomized controlled trial. *Schizophrenia Research*, *157*(1–3), 90–8.

Kirkpatrick, B., Fenton, W. S., Carpenter, W. T., and Marder, S. R. (2006). The NIMH-MATRICS consensus statement on negative symptoms. *Schizophrenia Bulletin* **32**(2), 214–19.

Klingberg, S., Wölwer, W., Engel, C., Wittorf, A., Herrlich, J., Meisner, C., et. al. (2011). Negative symptoms of schizophrenia as primary target of cognitive behavioral therapy: results of the randomized clinical TONES study. *Schizophrenia Bulletin*, *37*(S2), 98–110.

Kreyenbuhl, B., Buchanan, R.W., Dickerson, F. B., Dixon, L. B. (2010). The Schizophrenia Patient Outcomes Research Team (PORT): updated treatment recommendations 2009. *Schizophrenia Bulletin*, **36**(1), 94–103.

Kurtz, M. M., Mueser, K. T. (2008). A meta-analysis of controlled research on social skills training for schizophrenia. *Journal of Consulting and Clinical Psychology*, **76**, 491–504.

Kurtz, M. M., Richardson, C. L. (2012). Social cognitive training for schizophrenia: a meta-analytic investigation of controlled research. *Schizophrenia Bulletin*, **38**(5), 1092–104.

Kurtz, M. M., Gagen, E., Rocha, N. B., Machado, S., Penn, D. L. (2016). Comprehensive treatments for social cognitive deficits in schizophrenia: a critical review and effect-size analysis of controlled studies. *Clinical Psychology Review*, *43*, 80–9.

Laursen, T. M. (2011). Life expectancy among persons with schizophrenia or bipolar affective disorder. *Schizophrenia Research*, *131*(1–3), 101–4.

Leucht, S., Leucht, C., Huhn, M., Chaimani, A., Mavridis, D., Helfer, B., et al. (2017). Sixty years of placebo-controlled antipsychotic drug trials in acute schizophrenia: systematic review, Bayesian meta-analysis, and meta-regression of efficacy predictors. *American Journal of Psychiatry*, **174**(10), 927–42.

Loh, S. Y., Abdullah, A., Bakar, A. K. A., Thambu, M., Jaafar, N. R. N. (2016). Structured walking and chronic institutionalized schizophrenia inmates: a pilot RCT study on quality of life. *Global Journal of Health Science*, 8(1), 238–49.

Lutgens, D., Gariepy, G., Malla, A. (2017). Psychological and psychosocial interventions for negative symptoms in psychosis: systematic review and meta-analysis. *British Journal of Psychiatry*, **210**(5), 324–32.

Lysaker, P. H., Bell, M. D., Zito, W. S., Bioty, S. M. (1995) Social skills at work: Deficits and predictors of improvement in schizophrenia. *Journal of Nervous and Mental Disease*, *183*(11), 688–92.

McFarlane, W. R., Lukens, E., Link, B., Dushay, R., Deakins, S. A., Newmark, M., et al. (1995). Multiple family group and psychoeducation in the treatment of schizophrenia. *Archives of General Psychiatry*, **52**(8), 679–87.

McGurk, S. R., Twamley, E. W., Sitzer, D. I., McHugo, G. J., Mueser, K. T. (2007). A meta-analysis of cognitive remediation in schizophrenia. *American Journal of Psychiatry*, **164**, 1791–802.

Morrison, A.P. (2001). The interpretation of intrusions in psychosis: an integrative cognitive approach to hallucinations and delusions. *Behavioural and Cognitive Psychotherapy*, **29**(3), 257–76.

Mueser, K. T., Bellack, A. S. (1998). 'Social skills and social functioning' in K. T. Mueser and N. Tarrier (eds), *Handbook of Social Functioning in Schizophrenia*. Needham Heights, MA: Allyn & Bacon, pp. 79–96.

Mueser, K. T., Bellack, A. S., Douglas, M. S., Morrison, R. L. (1991). Prevalence and stability of social skill deficits in schizophrenia. *Schizophrenia Research*, 5(2), 167–76.

NCCMH (National Collaborating Centre for Mental Health). (2003). Schizophrenia. Full National Clinical Guideline on Core Interventions in Primary and Secondary Care. Royal College of Psychiatrists and the British Psychological Society.

NICE (National Institute for Health and Care Excellence) (2009). Schizophrenia: Core Interventions in the Treatment and Management of Schizophrenia in Adults in Primary and Secondary Care. CG82 (updated edition). London, The British Psychological Society and the Royal College of Psychiatrists.

Nuechterlein, K. H., Barch, D. M., Gold, J. M., Goldberg, T. E., Green, M. F., Heaton, R. K. (2004). Identification of separable cognitive factors in schizophrenia. *Schizophrenia Research*, 72(1), 29–39.

Nuechterlein, K. H., Ventura, J., McEwen, S. C., Gretchen-Doorly, D., Vinogradov, S., Subotnik, K. L. (2016). Enhancing cognitive training through aerobic exercise after a first schizophrenia episode: theoretical conception and pilot study. *Schizophrenia Bulletin*, **42**(suppl_1), S44–S52.

O'Reardon, J. P., Peshek, A. D., Romero, R., Cristancho, P. (2006). Neuromodulation and transcranial magnetic stimulation (TMS): a 21st century paradigm for therapeutics in psychiatry. *Psychiatry (Edgmont)*, **3**(I), 30–40.

Paulus, W. (2011). Transcranial electrical stimulation (tES–tDCS; tRNS, tACS) methods. *Neuropsychological Rehabilitation*, **21**(5), 602–17.

Payne, H. (1993). *Handbook of Inquiry in the Arts Therapies: One River, Many Currents*. London, Jessica Kingsley Publishers.

Petersen, L., Nordentoft, M., Jeppesen, P., Thorup, A., Christensen, T. Ø., Krarup, G., et al. (2005). Improving 1-year outcome in first-episode psychosis: OPUS trial. *British Journal of Psychiatry*, **187**(S48). s98–s103.

Priebe, S., Savill, M., Wykes, T., Bentall, R. P., Reininghaus, U., Lauber, C., et al. (2016). Effectiveness of group body psychotherapy for negative symptoms of schizophrenia: multicentre randomised controlled trial. *British Journal of Psychiatry*, **209**(1), 54–61.

Reeder, C., Wykes, T. (2010). *Cognitive Interaction Remediation of Cognition—a Training for Schizophrenia (CIRCuiTS)*. London, King's College London.

Romain, A. J., Fankam, C., Karelis, A. D., Letendre, E., Mikolajczak, G., Stip, E. et al. (2018). Effects of high intensity interval training among overweight individuals with psychotic disorders: a randomized controlled trial. *Schizophrenia Research*, *210*, 278–86.

Salzberg, S. (1995). *Loving-Kindness: The Revolutionary Art of Happiness*. Boston, Shambhala.

Scheewe, T. W., Backx, F. J. G., Takken, T., Jörg, F., Van Strater, A. C. P., Kroes, A., et al. (2013). Exercise therapy improves mental and physical health in schizophrenia: a randomised controlled trial. *Acta Psychiatrica Scandinavica*, *127*(6), 464–73.

Segal, Z. V., Teasdale, J. D., Williams, J. M. G. (2004). 'Mindfulness-based cognitive therapy: theoretical rationale and empirical status' in S. C. Hayes, V. M. Follette, M. M. Linehan (eds), *Mindfulness and Acceptance: Expanding the Cognitive-Behavioral Tradition*. New York, Guilford Press, pp. 45–65.

Stanford, A., Corcoran, C., Bulow, P., Bellovin-Weiss, S., Malaspina, D., Lisanby, S. H. (2011). High frequency prefrontal rTMS for the negative symptoms of schizophrenia: a case series. *Journal of ECT*, *27*, 11–7.

Strauss, G. P., Gold, J. M. (2012). A new perspective on anhedonia in schizophrenia. *American Journal of Psychiatry*, *169*(4), 364–73.

Staring, A. B., ter Huurne, M. A. B., van der Gaag, M. (2013). Cognitive behavioral therapy for negative symptoms (CBT-n) in psychotic disorders: a pilot study. *Journal of Behavior Therapy and Experimental Psychiatry*, *44*(3), 300–6.

Varambally, S., Gangadhar, B. N., Thirthalli, J., Jagannathan, A., Kumar, S., Venkatasubramanian, G., et al. (2012). Therapeutic efficacy of add-on yogasana intervention in stabilized outpatient schizophrenia: Randomized controlled comparison with exercise and waiting list. *Indian Journal of Psychiatry*, *54*(3), 227–32.

Velthorst, E., Koeter, M., Van Der Gaag, M., Nieman, D. H., Fett, A. K., Smit, F., et al. (2015). Adapted cognitive–behavioural therapy required for targeting negative symptoms in schizophrenia: meta-analysis and meta-regression. *Psychological Medicine*, *45*(3), 453–65.

Wassermann, E. M., Lisanby, S. H. (2001). Therapeutic application of repetitive transcranial magnetic stimulation: a review. *Clinical Neurophysiology*, *112*(8), 1367–77.

Wolkin, A., Sanfilipo, M., Wolf, A. P., Angrist, B., Brodie, J. D., and Rotrosen, J. (1992) Negative symptoms and hypofrontality in chronic schizophrenia' *Archives of General Psychiatry* **49**(12), 959–65.

Wykes, T., Steel, C., Everitt, B., Tarrier, N. (2008). Cognitive behavior therapy for schizophrenia: effect sizes, clinical models, and methodological rigor. *Schizophrenia Bulletin*, *34*(3), 523–37.

Wynne, L. (1988). 'An overview of the state of the art: What should be expected in current family therapy research' in L. Wynne (ed.), *The State of the Art in Family Therapy*

Research: Controversies and Recommendations. New York, Family Process Press, pp. 249–66.

Yamagata, T., Nakayama, Y., Tanji, J., Hoshi, E. (2012). Distinct information representation and processing for goal-directed behavior in the dorsolateral and ventrolateral prefrontal cortex and the dorsal premotor cortex. *Journal of Neuroscience*, **32**(37), 12934–49.

Scale for the Assessment of Negative Symptoms (SANS)

0 = None 1 = Questionable 2 = Mild 3 = Moderate 4 = Marked 5 = Severe	
Affective Fattening or Blunting	
1 *Unchanging facial expression.* The patient's face appears wooden, changes less than expected as emotional content of discourse changes.	0 1 2 3 4 5
2 *Decreased spontaneous movements.* The patient shows few or no spontaneous movements, does not shift position, move extremities, etc.	0 1 2 3 4 5
3 *Paucity of expressive gestures.* The patient does not use hand gestures, body position, etc., as an aid to expressing his ideas.	0 1 2 3 4 5
4 *Poor eye contact.* The patient avoids eye contact or "stares through" interviewer even when speaking.	0 1 2 3 4 5
5 *Affective nonresponsivity.* The patient fails to smile or laugh when prompted.	0 1 2 3 4 5
6 *Lack of vocal inflections.* The patients fails to show normal vocal emphasis patterns, is often monotonic.	0 1 2 3 4 5
7 *Global rating of affective flattening.* This rating should focus on overall severity of symptoms, especially unresponsiveness, eye contact, facial expression, and vocal inflections.	0 1 2 3 4 5
Alogia	
8 *Poverty of speech.* The patient's replies to questions are restricted in *amount* tend to be brief, concrete, and unelaborated.	0 1 2 3 4 5
9 *Poverty of content of speech.* The patient's replies are adequate in amount but tend to be vague, overconcrete, or overgeneralized, and convey little information.	0 1 2 3 4 5
10 *Blocking.* The patient indicates, either spontaneously or with prompting, that his [her] train of thought was interrupted.	0 1 2 3 4 5
11 *Increased latency of response.* The patient takes a long time to reply to questions; prompting indicates the patient is aware of the question.	0 1 2 3 4 5

12	*Global rating of alogia.* The core features of alogia are poverty of speech and poverty of content.	0 1 2 3 4 5
Avolition–Apathy		
13	*Grooming and hygiene* The patient's clothes may be sloppy or soiled, and he [she] may have greasy hair, body odor, etc.	0 1 2 3 4 5
14	*Impersistence at work or school* The patient has difficulty seeking or maintaining employment, completing schoolwork, keeping house, etc. If an inpatient, cannot persist at ward activities, such as occupational therapy, playing cards, etc.	0 1 2 3 4 5
15	*Physical anergia* The patient tends to be physically inert. He [she] may sit for hours and does not initiate spontaneous activity.	0 1 2 3 4 5
16	*Global rating of avolition–apathy* Strong weight may be given to one or two prominent symptoms if particularly striking.	0 1 2 3 4 5
Anhedonia–Asociality		0 1 2 3 4 5
17	*Recreational interests and activities* The patient may have few or no interests. Both the quality and quantity of interests should be taken into account.	0 1 2 3 4 5
18	*Sexual activity* The patient may show a decrease in sexual interest and activity, or enjoyment when active.	0 1 2 3 4 5
19	*Ability to feel intimacy and closeness* The patient may display an inability to form close or intimate relationships, especially with the opposite sex and family.	0 1 2 3 4 5
20	*Relationships with friends and peers* The patient may have few or no friends and may prefer to spend all of his [her] time isolated.	0 1 2 3 4 5
21	*Global rating of anhedonia–asociality* This rating should reflect overall severity, taking into account the patient's age, family status, etc.	0 1 2 3 4 5
Attention		
22	*Social inattentiveness* The patient appears uninvolved or unengaged. He [she] may seem spacey.	0 1 2 3 4 5
23	*Inattentiveness during mental status testing* Test of "serial 7s" (at least five subtractions) and spelling *world* backward. Score: 2 = 1 error; 3 = 2 errors; 4 = 3 errors.	0 1 2 3 4 5
24	*Global rating of attention* This rating should assess the patient's overall concentration, clinically and on tests.	0 1 2 3 4 5

Negative Symptom Assessment-16 (NSA-16) Rating Scale—Short Form

1. Prolonged time to respond
   1) no abnormal pauses before speaking
   2) minimal evidence of inappropriate pauses, may be extreme of normal
   3) occasional long pauses before answering questions
   4) pauses occur frequently (20–40% of responses)
   5) pauses occur most of the time (40–80% of responses)
   6) pauses occur with almost every response (80–100% of responses)
   9) not ratable (use only when all efforts to rate this item have failed)

2. Restricted speech quantity
   1) normal speech quantity
   2) minimal reduction in quantity, may be extreme of normal
   3) speech quantity is reduced, but more obtained with minimal prodding
   4) flow of speech is maintained only by regularly prodding
   5) responses usually limited to a few words, and/or detail is only obtained by prodding or bribing
   6) responses usually nonverbal or limited to 1 or 2 words, despite efforts to elicit more
   9) not ratable (use only when all efforts to rate this item have failed)

3. Impoverished speech content
   1) normal speech content
   2) minimal reduction in content, may be extreme of normal
   3) ideas are sometimes vague
   4) many ideas vague; some ideas remain vague, even after attempts to clarify
   5) most ideas remain vague, even after attempts to clarify
   6) no ideas can be clarified beyond vague impressions
   9) not ratable (use only when all efforts to rate this item have failed)

4. Inarticulate speech
   1) speech clear, not mumbled
   2) minimal garbled speech, may be extreme or normal
   3) a few words are slurred, but can be understood in context
   4) the subject must occasionally be asked to repeat mumbled words
   5) many words are difficult to understand; the subject must frequently be asked to repeat but, on repeating, can usually be understood
   6) little language can be understood even after repeating
   9) not ratable (use only when all efforts to rate this item have failed)

5. Emotion: Reduced range (specify time frame for this assessment)
   1) normal range of emotion
   2) minimal reduction in range, may be extreme of normal
   3) range seems restricted relative to a normal person, but during the specified time period subject convincingly reports at least 4 emotions
   4) subject convincingly identifies 2 or 3 emotional experiences

5) subject can convincingly identify only 1 emotional experience
6) subject reports little or no emotional range
9) not ratable (use only when all efforts to rate this item have failed)

6. Affect: Reduced modulation of intensity
   1) normal modulation of affect
   2) minimal reduction of modulation, may be extreme or normal
   3) affective intensity is muted relative to normal, but some spontaneous change in affective intensity appropriate to the content of conversation is observed
   4) affective responses are clearly blunted, but by asking more pointed questions, appropriate changes in affective intensity can be elicited
   5) intensity of affect is modulated only slightly, even after prodding
   6) affective responses are never modulated, even after prodding
   9) not ratable (use only when all efforts to rate this item have failed)

7. Affect: Reduced display on demand
   1) subject convincingly displays all requested affective expressions
   2) subject convincingly displays 5 of the 6 requested affective expressions
   3) subject displays any 4 of the 6 requested affective expressions
   4) subject displays any 2 or 3 of the 6 requested affective expressions
   5) subject displays any 1 of the 6 requested affective expressions
   6) subject is unable to display any requested affective expression
   9) not ratable (use only when all efforts to rate this item have failed)

8. Reduced social drive
   1) normal social drive
   2) minimal reduction in social drive, may be extreme of normal
   3) desire for social interactions seems somewhat reduced
   4) obvious reduction in desire to initiate social contacts, but a number of social contacts are initiated each week
   5) marked reduction in desire to initiate social contacts, but a few contacts are maintained at subject's initiation (as with family)
   6) no desire to initiate any social interactions
   9) not ratable (use only when all efforts to rate this item have failed)

9. Poor rapport with interviewer
   1) normal rapport
   2) minimal reduction in rapport, may be extreme of normal
   3) interviewer sometimes has to carry the conversation because the subject's interest seems reduced
   4) interchanges are generally dull and uninspiring; interviewer must often lead the conversation because subject is detached
   5) interviewer must prod to engage the subject in the interview
   6) prodding does not result in engagement with the interviewer
   9) not ratable (use only when all efforts to rate this item have failed)

10. Interest in emotional and physical intimacy
   1) desires to engage in some form of emotional and physical intimacy once a day or more
   2) desires to engage in some form of emotional and physical intimacy 3–6 times a week
   3) desires to engage in some form of emotional and physical intimacy once or twice a week
   4) desires to engage in some form of emotional and physical intimacy 1–3 times a month
   5) desires to engage in some form of emotional and physical intimacy several times a year
   6) no desire for emotional and physical intimacy is reported
   9) not ratable (use only when all efforts to rate this item have failed)

11. Poor grooming and hygiene
   1) normal grooming and hygiene
   2) minimally reduced grooming and hygiene, may be extreme of normal
   3) clean but untidy, or clothes are mismatched
   4) clothes are unkempt or unbuttoned (looks as if subject just got out of bed)
   5) clothes are dirty or stained, or subject has an odor
   6) clothes are badly soiled and/or subject has a foul odor
   9) not ratable (use only when all efforts to rate this item have failed)

12. Reduced sense of purpose
   1) normal sense of purpose
   2) minimal reduction in purpose, may be extreme of normal
   3) life goals somewhat vague, but current activities suggest purpose
   4) subject has difficulty coming up with life goals, but activities are directed toward limited goal or goals
   5) goals are very limited or have to be suggested, and activities are not focused toward achieving any of them
   6) no identifiable life goals
   9) not ratable (use only when all efforts to rate this item have failed)

13. Reduced interests
   1) normal interests
   2) minimal reduction in interests, may be extreme of normal
   3) range of interests and/or commitment to them seems diminished
   4) range of interests is clearly diminished and subject is not particularly committed to interests held
   5) only 1 or 2 interests reported, and these pursued superficially
   6) little or nothing stimulates interest
   9) not ratable (use only when all efforts to rate this item have failed)

14. Reduced daily activity
    1) normal daily activity
    2) minimal reduction in activity, may be extreme of normal
    3) employed, attends school or volunteers, but is underachieving; few hobbies
    4) not involved in the activities expected of a normal young person (may be unemployed, or minimally employed for education, but he may be involved in mental health program one or more days a week)
    5) most of day spent doing things that require minimal mental or physical exertion (watches TV, smokes, drinks coffee, walks to store, but he may be involved in a mental health program one or more days a week)
    6) most of day is spent sitting in a chair or lying in bed; has little or no regard for what goes on in immediate environment
    9) not ratable (use only when all efforts to rate this item have failed)

15. Reduced expressive gestures
    1) normal expressive gestures
    2) minimal reduction in gestures, may be extreme of normal
    3) hand and head gestures normally seen during conversation are reduced
    4) hand or head gestures are infrequent; gestures may be limited to periods when the subject is discussing topics of special interest to him
    5) gestures infrequent even during discussion of highly emotional topics
    6) gestures are never observed
    9) not ratable (use only when all efforts to rate this item have failed)

16. Slowed movements
    1) normal speed of movements
    2) minimal reduction in speed of movements, may be extreme of normal
    3) voluntary movements are slightly retarded or slowed
    4) movements are generally sluggish
    5) most movements are retarded and made with effort
    6) all movements are made with extreme effort; subject must be assisted from chair
    9) not ratable (use only when all efforts to rate this item have failed)

Global Negative Symptoms Rating

1. No evidence of this symptom
2. Minimal evidence of this symptom
3. Mild evidence of this symptom
4. Moderate evidence of this symptom, apparent to the casual observer
5. Marked evidence of this symptom, readily apparent to casual observer
6. Severe, not only obvious but has marked impact on functioning
7. Extremely severe symptom, it is incapacitating for subject

Reproduced from Negative Symptom Assessment-16 (NSA-16) Instruction Manual, Version 1.1, Larry Alphs. ©2006 with the kind permission from Dr Larry Alphs.

Negative Symptom Assessment-4 (NSA-4)

Definition

Negative symptoms represent the reduction or absence of behaviors normally present in a healthy person. These include, but are not limited to, behaviors related to personal, social and affective behavior. Specifically, negative symptoms of schizophrenia are considered to include reduction in emotional expression and perception, reduction in the fluency and productivity of thought and speech, reduced desire for social involvement and reduced social interaction with others and a loss or lack of goal-directed behavior. These symptoms contribute to substantial reductions in the functioning of schizophrenic patients as compared to others in their society.

1. Restricted speech quantity

This item assesses the amount of speech the subject provides in the course of the interview. Ratings on this item suggest that the subject gives brief answers to questions and/or provides elaborating details only after the interviewer prods him.

1. Normal speech quantity
2. Minimal reduction in quantity, may be extreme of normal
3. Speech seems reduced, but more can be obtained with minimal prodding
4. Speech is maintained only by regularly prodding the subject
5. Responses are usually limited to a few words and/or details are only obtained by prodding or bribing
6. Responses are usually non-verbal or limited to 1 or 2 word answers (despite one's best efforts to get the subject to elaborate)
9. Not ratable (use only when all efforts to rate this item have failed)

2. Emotion: Reduced range (specify time frame for this assessment)

Emotion is the feeling content of a person's inner life. This item assesses the range of emotion experienced by the subject during the last week (or other specified time period). Base ratings on the subject's answers to queries of whether he/she has felt happy, sad, etc. during the last week, as well as any reports of having these emotions later in the interview. A full range of emotions would include, but not be limited to happiness, sadness, pride, fear, surprise, and anger. This item should be distinguished from the capacity to display affect, which is rated elsewhere. (If you sense that a subject's emotional life is autistic and not contextually validated, rate his/her emotional range according to your interpretations of his/her experience.)

1. Normal range of emotion
2. Minimal reduction in range, may be extreme of normal
3. Range seems restricted relative to a normal person, but during the specified time frame subject convincingly reports at least 4 emotions.
4. Subject convincingly identifies 2 or 3 emotional experiences
5. Subject convincingly identifies only 1 emotional experience
6. Subject reports little or no emotional range
9. Not ratable (use only when all efforts to rate this item have failed)

3. Reduced social drive

This item assesses how much the subject <u>desires</u> to initiate social interactions. Desire may be measured in part by the number of actual or attempted social contacts with others. To rate severity probes the type of social interactions, and their frequency. Remember the reference range is a normal 20 year old. Many subjects may be rated 2 to 3.

1. normal social drive
2. minimal reduction in social drive, may be extreme of normal
3. desire for social interactions seems somewhat reduced
4. obvious reduction in desire to initiate social contacts, but a number of social contacts are initiated each week
5. marked reduction in desire to initiate social contacts, but a few contacts are maintained at subject's initiation (as with family)
6. no desire to initiate any social interactions
9. not ratable (use only when all efforts to rate this item have failed)

4. Reduced interests

This item assesses the range and intensity of the subject's interests.

1. Normal interests
2. Minimal reduction in interests, may be extreme of normal
3. Range of interests and/or commitment to them seems diminished
4. Range of interests is clearly diminished and is not particularly committed to interests held
5. Only 1 or 2 interests reported, and these pursued superficially
6. No identifiable goals
9. Not ratable (use only when all efforts to rate this item have failed)

Global Rating

1. No evidence of this symptom
2. Minimal evidence of this symptom
3. Mild evidence of this symptom
4. Moderate evidence of this symptom, apparent to the casual observer
5. Marked evidence of this symptom, readily apparent to casual observer
6. Severe, not only obvious but has marked impact on functioning
7. Extremely severe symptom, it is incapacitating for subject

Reproduced from Negative Symptom Assessment-4 (NSA-4) Manual Version 1.0
Larry Alphs. ©2006 with the kind permission from Dr Larry Alphs.

Brief negative symptom scale (BNSS)

List of the items

1. INTENSITY OF PLEASURE DURING ACTIVITIES
2. FREQUENCY OF PLEASURABLE ACTIVITIES
3. INTENSITY OF EXPECTED PLEASURE FROM FUTURE ACTIVITIES
4. LACK OF NORMAL DISTRESS

5. ASOCIALITY: BEHAVIOR
6. ASOCIALITY: INTERNAL EXPERIENCE
7. AVOLITION: BEHAVIOR
8. AVOLITION: INTERNAL EXPERIENCE
9. FACIAL EXPRESSION
10. VOCAL EXPRESSION
11. EXPRESSIVE GESTURES
12. QUANTITY OF SPEECH
13. SPONTANEOUS ELABORATION

Examples of probe questions for selected items

Probe questions for anticipatory anhedonia (Item 3):

If the subject did enjoy some activities over the past week: *You said you en-joyed . . . (based on the interview). Do you expect to do any of those again soon?*
If Yes: *How do you think you'll feel when you do that? Are you looking forward to it?*
If No: *Do you want to do that again? Is there something else you would enjoy doing? (If yes: How do you think you'll feel when you do that?)*
If the subject did not enjoy any activities in the past week: *Are there any activities that you are looking forward to? Is there anything else you'd look forward to doing?*

Probe questions for Avolition: Behavior (Item 7)

General: *Tell me how you spend your time. Do you spend much time just sitting, not doing anything in particular?*
Work and school:
If currently working or going to school:
Did you make it to work (or school) this week? How much time did you spend working (or in school or studying)? Do you get there on your own? Do you wait for others to tell you what to do, or do you start the work (or schoolwork) yourself?
If not currently working or going to school:
Have you looked for work or looked into taking classes in the past week? Did someone suggest it, or did you do that on your own?
If Yes: *What did you do?*
If No: *Why not? [Ask to distinguish opportunity from motivation]*

Item 7 has further probe question about 'Recreation/hobbies/pastimes' and 'Self-care'.

Probe questions for Avolition: Internal Experience (Item 8)

Probe Questions
Work and school:

If currently working or going to school: *Is your job (or school) is important to you? Do you think about it much? Do you feel motivated about it?*
If not working or going to school: *Do you think about getting a job or going to school? Do you miss having a job (or going to school)?*

If Yes: *What did you do?*

If No: *Why not? [Ask to distinguish opportunity from motivation]*

Recreation/Hobbies/Pastimes: What do you do in your free time? *What hobbies do you have? Were you thinking about these this week?*

Self-care: *Did you feel motivated to take care of yourself this week? (If an explanation is needed: motivated about bathing, cleaning your home, taking care of your health, etc.)*

If Yes: *How so?*

Index

Note: Tables, figures and boxes are indicated by *t*, *f* and *b* following the page number.

Schmidt, S. J. 21, 22
Schneider, J. K. 52
Schneider, K. 3
Schooler, N. R. 100
Schulte, P. F. 76, 77
Schultze-Lutter, F. 20, 21, 22, 23b,
    25, 26, 27b, 29, 30
Scorza, F. A. 80
secondary negative symptoms
    1–2, 40
    and basic symptoms 21, 22,
        23b, 27b, 33
    case vignette 7b
    classification 6–9
    course of schizophrenia 10, 11f
    long-term course 41f
    pharmacologic treatment
        69, 71, 81
        antipsychotics 72, 73
    self-evaluation 51, 59–63
second-generation antipsychotics
    (SGAs) 68, 70, 71,
    72, 74, 81
second-rank symptoms 3
Seddighi, S. 77
Segal, Z. V. 93
selective serotonin reuptake
    inhibitors (SSRIs) 75
Self-Assessment Anhedonia Scale
    (SAAS) 60t, 61–2
self-disturbances 20
self-evaluation 4, 51–63
    primary negative
        symptoms 53–9
    secondary negative
        symptoms 59–63
        anhedonia 59–62
        apathy 62
        psychiatric experiences 59
Self-evaluation of Negative
    Symptoms (SNS)
    54–9, 57t
self-presentation,
    disturbance in 27b
Self-reported Apathy Evaluation
    Scale (AES-S) 60t, 62
Selten, J. P. 52, 54
Sepehry, A. A. 75
D-serine 76, 77
sertindole 72
Sevy, S. 55
sex hormones 80–1, 82
Shapiro, S. 93
Shaw, J. 87
Shen, Y. 79
Shilling, P. D. 80
Short, R. A. 96
Sijben, N. E. 54
Silva, M. J. 80
Silver, H. 75
Simonsen, C. 62
simvastatin 80
Singh, J. 78
Singh, S. P. 76, 77
Singh, V. 76, 77
Sisti, D. 81
Sitzer, D. I. 89
skills training 88t, 90–1, 99

Slooff, C. J. 78
Smirnis, N. K. 59
Smith, J. D. 76
Smulevich, A. B. 40, 41, 42,
    44, 45, 47
Snezhnevsky, A. V. 42, 48
Social and Occupational
    Functioning Assessment
    Scale 25
Social Anhedonia Scale (SAS)
    60t, 61
    Revised (R-SAS) 61
social attention, disturbances of/
    social inattentiveness 6
social deprivation/disadvantage,
    negative symptoms
    secondary to 8–9
social skills training 88t, 90–1, 99
social withdrawal see asociality
Solli, H. P. 96
speech
    abnormalities, as fundamental
        symptoms 40
    disturbance of expressive 23b
    disturbance of receptive 23b
Spring, B. 79
Spuch, C. 79
Stahl, D. 70, 99
Stanford, A. D. 76, 94
Staring, A. B. 92
statins 79–80
Steel, C. 92
Stefanics, G. 6
Stefanis, N. C. 59
Steinmeyer, E. M. 22, 25
Stepner, M. 9
stereotyped thinking 6
stimulants 75–6
Stip, E. 75
Strauss, G. P. 14, 52, 56, 69, 89
stress tolerance, impaired 27b
Strosahl, K. D. 93
Structured Interview for
    Psychosis-Risk Syndromes
    (SIPS) 31, 32–3
Subjective Deficit Syndrome Scale
    (SDSS) 53
Subjective Experience of
    Deficits in Schizophrenia
    (SEDS) 53
Subjective Experience of
    Negative Symptoms
    (SENS) 54, 59
subjective experiences
    asociality 5
    evaluation 4
    self-evaluation 53–4, 59
    substance use 8
Sullivan, K. M. 79
Süllwold, L. 25
sulpiride 73
Summerfelt, A. 13
Susser, E. 75
Switch trials 70

T

Tajik-Esmaeeli, S. 80

Takken, T. 97
Tanji, J. 94
Tarbox, S. I. 30
Taylor, K. N. 93
Taylor, M. J. 25
Taylor, S. F. 62
Teasdale, J. D. 93
Temporal Experience of Pleasure
    Scale (TEPS) 60t, 62
Teng, B. L. 80
Ter Huurne, M. A. B. 92
Thaker, G. 61
Thal, L. J. 78
Theodoridou, A. 20, 21
Thibaut, F. 41
thinking, slowness in 27b
Thirthalli, J. 97
thought blockages 23b
thought energy, lack of 27b
thought interference 23b, 30
thought perseveration 23b, 30
thought pressure 23b
Tiihonen, J. 76, 78
topiramate 78
transcranial direct current
    stimulation (tDCS) 94, 95
trema 26
Trimble, M. R. 41
Trower, P. 92
true memories/fantasy,
    decreased ability to
    discriminate between
    =basic symptoms 23b, 30
Tso, I. F. 62
Tuominen, H. J. 76
Twamley, E. W. 89
Type I schizophrenia 9
Type II schizophrenia 9

U

Üçok, A. 10, 40
United States
    FDA see Food and Drug
        Administration (FDA), US
    NIMH see National Institute
        for Mental Health
        (NIMH), US
Upthegrove, R. 55
Usall, J. 80
Ushakov, U. V. 41

V

valproate 78
Van Den Bosch, R. J. 52, 54
Van Der Gaag, M. 92
van der Most, P. J. 79
Varambally, S. 97
Veerman, S. R. 76, 77, 78
Velligan, D. I. 67
Velthorst, E. 88t, 92, 93
Ventura, J. 99
Vignapiano, A. 14, 56
Virdee, G. 89
visual field, captivation of
    attention by details of
    the 23b